Texas College
of
Osteopathic Medicine

Texas College of Osteopathic Medicine

༄༅ *The First Twenty Years*

Collected and Edited by
C. Ray Stokes

Text by
Judy Alter

Texas College of Osteopathic Medicine
with
The University of North Texas Press

Copyright © 1990, Texas College of Osteopathic Medicine

Library of Congress Cataloging-in-Publication Data

Texas College of Osteopathic Medicine : the first twenty years /
    collected and edited by C. Ray Stokes ; text by Judy Alter.
        p.   cm.
    ISBN 0-929398-17-3
    1. Texas College of Osteopathic Medicine—History.   2. Osteopathic
schools—Texas—History.   I. Stokes, C. Ray.   II. Alter, Judy,
1938–
    [DNLM: 1. Texas College of Osteopathic Medicine.   2. Osteopathic
Medicine—education.   3. Schools, Medical—history—Texas.   W 19
T3548]
RZ338.U6T48   1990
610'.71'1764—dc20
DNLM/DLC
for Library of Congress   90-10946
                                                                               CIP

Photo Credits: With the following exceptions, all photographs are from the Texas College of
Osteopathic Medicine archives. The photo on page 16 is from the Rhea-Engert Studio, Fort
Worth; on 18 by Thomas R. Turner, D.O., Fort Worth; on 22 and 98 by Bill Wood, Fort
Worth; on 47, 49, 62, and 74, the University of North Texas archives, Denton; on 55 by Bill
Malone, Austin; on 65 and 67 by Paul Talley, Dallas; on 88 (top) courtesy *Fort Worth
Star-Telegram*; and on 113 by Randall Photography, Arlington.

Additional copies of *Texas College of Osteopathic Medicine* can be ordered through University
Press Distributors, Drawer C, College Station, Texas 77843. TCOM is located at Camp
Bowie Boulevard and Montgomery Street, Forth Worth, Texas 76107.

This book was designed by A. Tracy Row.
Manufactured in the USA.

Contents

Dedication

To the Texas College of Osteopathic Medicine's founders with affection and admiration:

George J. Luibel, D.O., FAAO
Dan D. Beyer, D.O.
Carl E. Everett, D.O.

༂༂ *Foreword*

". . . A MAN'S REACH SHOULD EXCEED HIS GRASP, OR WHAT'S A
HEAVEN FOR?"

—Robert Browning

George J. Luibel, D.O., seemed to fit the mold of Browning's
immortal words, reaching farther than anyone thought he could
grasp, when he sparked the unlikely birth of the seventh existing
osteopathic college in the United States. But with the help of
D. D. Beyer, D.O., and Carl E. Everett, D.O., he did just that. This
thin volume, based heavily on reminiscent accounts, is testimony to
the first twenty years of the Texas College of Osteopathic Medicine
and to George Luibel's reach.

TCOM's brief history has been chronicled several times, including
a ten-year report in 1980 by Janice Odom, then public information
director, and Verlie McAlister, assistant, and a short history to be
published in the forthcoming *Handbook of Texas* (the new edition is
projected for 1995) that features the image and identity of the institution. This 1990 review of the past and future of a growing
medical college is not meant to be a text. Rather it is informal in
tone at the request and challenge to this writer by President David
M. Richards, D.O., and is intended as a celebration of the school's
twentieth anniversary and convocation.

Dr. Richards' challenge was accepted, but it could not have been
carried out without support. Many from the founding faculty, staff

XI

and early "TCOM family" came forward to record their memories and provide ideas and help. Judy Alter, award-winning Fort Worth author who was born into the "D.O. family," agreed to craft the text based on the memoirs and published sources compiled by this correspondent. This volume is the result.

Much editorial assistance should be credited to the executive committee and to the full editorial board. We are forever grateful to all of them. They are:

Craig S. Elam, M.L.S., associate director for technical services, Health Sciences Library; Bill Hix, manager of news and information; Mary Lu Schunder, Ph.D., associate professor of anatomy; Mark A. Baker, D.O. (TCOM Class of 1976), radiology department, Osteopathic Medical Center of Texas, Fort Worth; Carl E. Everett, D.O.; Diana Finley, associate director, Texas Osteopathic Medical Association; Roy B. Fisher, D.O., surgeon; Ben G. Harris, Ph.D., professor of biochemistry and associate dean of research; Elizabeth F. Harris, Ph.D., associate professor of microbiology and immunology; Robert L. Kaman, Ph.D., associate professor of public health and preventive medicine; Irvin M. Korr, Ph.D., professor of manipulative medicine; George J. Luibel, D.O.; and C. Raymond Olson, D. O., professor of medicine.

The fruition of this endeavor, however, goes beyond the merits of the editorial board and other contributors. It belongs to the first graduating class, which made it all possible. The eighteen members of the Class of '74 have set an excellent example of what determination can accomplish.

C. Ray Stokes
Curator of Special Collections
and College Historian
Fort Worth, January, 1990

ᔕᔐᔕ *Introduction*

"NOBODY EVER KNOWS AFTER IT BECOMES REAL HISTORY EX-
actly when that history really began." Those are the words of Dr.
Henry Hardt, founding dean of the Texas College of Osteopathic
Medicine, reflecting in 1982 on the history of the college. When did
TCOM begin? With an idea in someone's mind? Out of a committee
action expressing a need for more osteopathic colleges? Perhaps in
Labor Day weekend meetings between physicians and longtime
friends? Maybe with the opening some thirty years earlier of a small,
struggling osteopathic hospital? All of these threads and more were
woven together to create the Texas College of Osteopathic Medicine as it stands today.

TCOM came into being in large part because of the hard work of
three osteopathic physicians and their refusal to be discouraged by
what seemed an impossible task. George Luibel, Carl Everett and
D. D. "Danny" Beyer simply didn't believe it couldn't be done.
With strong support from national, state and local osteopathic associations, they turned their dream into a reality. And on October
1, 1970, TCOM opened its doors. Appropriately enough, those rented
doors were on the fifth floor of the Fort Worth Osteopathic Hospital
(now known as Osteopathic Medical Center of Texas).

Even during the planning years, the college attracted dedicated
personnel—a public relations professional who became the college's
first employee, a chemistry professor who brought great expertise in
administrative matters and a needed familiarity with the Texas State

I

Board of Examiners in the Basic Sciences, basic scientists who became faculty members (even maintenance men when the need arose) and physicians who volunteered their time and donated books to the library.

The early years of the college were years of challenge laced with humor and fellowship. There was, always, a sense of working together for a goal—the growth of the college—and there was that togetherness that bonds people facing a challenge. Those who were involved in the early years of TCOM have, almost without exception, found their lives dramatically altered by the experience. Said one early faculty member, "Those were the most challenging, rewarding, happiest years of my professional career."

Progress came with time—an affiliation with North Texas State University (now the University of North Texas), acceptance as a state institution, remarkable growth of the physical plant, development of a viable research program, publication of a goals statement stressing preventive medicine and therefore unique to medical education. With progress came new faces, new contributors to the fabric that is TCOM. But, amazingly, many of the original builders and planners remain. Together, the old-timers and the newcomers have built a medical school of unusual dedication and purpose.

TCOM is today an institution which boasts a fifteen-acre campus on a hilltop with a breathtaking view of downtown Fort Worth. Its neighbors in the renowned cultural district are museums distinguished by their buildings, their collections and their reputations.

TCOM may be the newest kid on the block, but the institution fits into this neighborhood. Its three main buldings, all built since 1976, create a small skyline of their own within the city, a complex of modern design that speaks of a forward-looking and growing institution. Yet TCOM is much more than a collection of modern buildings.

It was Dr. Hardt who also said, "Few people have the opportunity to build a medical school." With those words, he captured the spirit of a unique and exhilarating experience shared by the men and women whose work created the college, whose dedication kept it going in the early, lean years, and whose persistence is rewarded today by the existence of a progressive and outstanding college of osteopathic medicine.

Today, TCOM is known not by its buildings but by its people—the doctors it has sent out to serve Texas and the United States, the faculty who teach within its walls, the students who study there. As the college approaches its twentieth anniversary, TCOM has an alumni body of over a thousand, a faculty of over 150, a staff of some 550, and a student body of nearly 400.

This, then, is the history of the first twenty years of an osteopathic medical college: a school dedicated to teaching wellness as a way of life; an institution devoted to being in the forefront of medicine as health, not just the treatment of disease.

This history is based on oral accounts compiled by Ray Stokes of TCOM. Because of Ray's dedicated work, the story of the school is told in the words of the people who built the college and lived its history.

Judy Alter
Fort Worth, January 1990

෪෪ *A Paper College*

THE COMMITTEE TO INVESTIGATE THE FEASIBILITY OF ESTAB-lishing an Osteopathic Medical School in Texas was formed in 1961 by the Texas Osteopathic Medical Association (TOMA) in response to an American Osteopathic Association (AOA) concern about the national need for more osteopathic physicians. There were at that time five osteopathic colleges, none of them in the Southwest. But at first much of the Texas committee's work concerned securing appropriations from the state for tuition grants for Texas students enrolled in osteopathic medical schools outside the state.

Beyond that, "the annual effort of that committee," recalls Dr. George Luibel, "would usually be to have a thirty-minute, more or less, meeting in somebody's hotel room, prior to the midyear meeting of the board of trustees, and then report to the board of trustees that the committee was still interested in this project."

In 1965, when Luibel was head of the committee, a list of recommendations was forwarded to the board of the state organization. The recommendations were: to establish a foundation to accept donations of money and land for the school; to hire an expert in medical education to survey the state and recommend a site for the school; to include in any planning the possibility of becoming part of an existing educational institution; to explore the possibility of moving an existing college of osteopathic medicine to Texas; to establish the college in an area where suitable teaching facilities and qualified clinicians were available; to seek substantial initial contributions "to get the ball rolling."

When the TOMA board took no action on the recommendations, Luibel's committee suggested that the committee be disbanded. Luibel says that by 1965 he had about decided that at the rate of progress then in effect the project would never get off the ground. "It was something everybody liked to talk about, but nobody really wanted to take the bull by the horns." Luibel suggests that this reticence was due to inexperience; the five existing osteopathic colleges had all been in operation for more than forty years, and there was no current example to follow in building a new college. An effort was underway at that time to build the Michigan College of Osteopathic Medicine, and Luibel was familiar with that project because of his position on the board of trustees of the AOA.

When the AOA board was asked to vote financial support to the proposed Michigan College of Osteopathic Medicine, which eventually opened a year before TCOM, Luibel told them, "I just want to put you all on notice that I'm going to come back and ask you for some money for a Texas college some day." And that's exactly what he did.

Dr. Roy Fisher remembers Labor Day weekends when several Fort Worth osteopathic physicians and their wives—the Luibels, the Everetts, the Danny Beyers, the Fishers—would get together at the Western Hills Motel coffee shop to talk about what could be done to open a college of osteopathic medicine in Texas. They felt strongly that Fort Worth was the logical site for such a school. The only major city in Texas without a medical school, it boasted the largest osteopathic hospital in the state and the largest collection of specialty physicians available for teaching purposes, and it was home to TOMA headquarters.

Fort Worth Osteopathic Hospital (FWOH) was then and is now essential to the existence of the college. The hospital—known from 1981 to 1989 as the Fort Worth Osteopathic Medical Center (FWOMC) but renamed the Osteopathic Medical Center of Texas early in 1990—was begun in an old mansion, now unfortunately demolished, on Summit Avenue, then still known by its turn-of-the-century name, "Silk Stocking Row." Fisher and his family lived on the second floor of the house; the hospital, with two beds at first and eventually twelve, occupied the ground floor. The institution was first called Fisher Hospital, because it was founded by Fisher and his brother, Dr. Ray Fisher; in 1946 the hospital was incorporated as Fort Worth Osteopathic Hospital. The staff of thirteen physicians included Drs. Luibel, Everett and Beyer, the three who later became college founders.

The hospital moved from the mansion on Summit Avenue to a twenty-five-bed facility in the 3600 block of Camp Bowie Boulevard in 1951 and then in 1956 built at its present location on Montgomery Street. The land on Montgomery was gained for the location of a hospital through the efforts of Dr. Phil Russell, known to osteopathic physicians and politicians throughout the state as "Mr. Osteopathy of Texas." Russell was the personal physician of *Fort Worth Star-Telegram* publisher Amon G. Carter, Sr., an association which founded a strong and important link between the Carter Foundation and the osteopathic profession. Carter, often called "Mr. Fort Worth" because of his civic enthusiasm, was an ardent advocate of osteopathic medicine due to the care given him by Dr. Russell. Oilman Sid Richardson was another patient of Russell's and a close friend of Carter's, and the Sid Richardson Foundation also contributed generously to the new hospital. In addition to these private donations, the hospital received the first Hill-Burton governmental funds granted an osteopathic institution in Texas.

In the spring of 1966, with a recommendation to disband the college committee pending before the TOMA board, rumors began to float that the College of Osteopathic Medicine and Surgery in Des Moines, Iowa, was considering moving to a new location because of a lack of support in Des Moines. The Texans invited officials of the Iowa college to come to Fort Worth for a visit. TOMA officals secured the support of the Council on Development of the Fort Worth Chamber of Commerce and actively began to seek a sixty-acre site for the medical school, should it relocate in Texas. Officials of the Des Moines college made not one but several trips

7

to Texas, and during one of those visits, a Des Moines dean posed the interesting dilemma of how the Iowa college would operate without a Texas charter.

"I told them we could get a charter, if that was all the problem was," says Luibel, "but I never figured they'd move. When people in Des Moines got wind of the fact that they were losing a stable institution that had been around since before the turn of the century, they were certainly going to do something to keep it there." They did, and the Des Moines college did not move in spite of an official invitation from TOMA, accompanied by an appropriation of $75,000 to initiate the move. But the encounter with the Des Moines college had revitalized interest, and Luibel saw the need for a charter in Texas.

In New York, an institution was required to have $300,000 in assets before the state would grant a charter; in Michigan, it was $100,000. In Texas, there was no monetary consideration, and Fort Worth lawyer Abe Herman, whose firm represented both the Carter publishing interests and Texas Christian University, assured Luibel that the cost of obtaining a charter would not be astronomical. "I was sitting and talking to my wife one night," Luibel remembers, "and I said, 'I just wonder who I could get to go in on a deal like that with me?' And I thought a few minutes and said, 'I believe I know who will do that.'"

Luibel called Carl Everett and Danny Beyer, and the three of them contributed about six hundred dollars expense money each to send Herman to Austin. He returned with the perpetual charter authorizing the Texas College of Osteopathic Medicine to grant the D.O. degree for the practice of osteopathic medicine and also the M.S. and such other scientific and honorary degrees as may be desirable. The charter also authorized such other facilities as nursing and medical technology schools and authorized the college to elect from three to twenty directors. The charter specified the City of Fort Worth as the site of the college and named the initial directors: Luibel, Everett and Beyer.

The three founders were in business. Between themselves, they named the officers of the non-profit corporation: Luibel was chairman; Everett, secretary-treasurer; and Beyer, vice chairman. Luibel suspects he was chairman because the other two didn't want to do all the running around and work he would have to do; Everett, however, credits Luibel's drive and connections with the success of the early college effort. Luibel had been active in professional politics and had long had an interest in the college project, so it was natural that he was both founder and chairman. Why did Beyer and Everett join him? Basically because Luibel asked them to. Both were family physcians with established practices in Fort Worth, and both were colleagues and close personal friends of Luibel.

Dr. John Burnett, a well-established general practitioner from the Dallas area, was elected as a fourth member of the board. He was followed by fellow Texans Dr. Sam Ganz of Corpus Christi, Dr. H. George Grainger of Tyler, Dr. John L. Witt of Groom, Dr. Glen Kumm of Portland, Dr. Michael Calabrese of El Paso, Dr. James Fite of Bonham, and Dr. Walters R. Russell of Dallas.

At that point, the new board had a paper college, but they had no business. "Now that we had the thing," said Luibel, "what were we going to do with it?"

One of the things Luibel did was to talk with an assistant to the Commissioner of Higher Education in the State of Texas. In a moment of candor, that official said, "I probably shouldn't tell you this, but I think if you are going to start a college, you ought to do it and then, if you want any state support, come and try to get it afterwards. If you try to get state funds to start your school, you'll be ten years ever getting off the launching pad."

The next step was to apply to the AOA for a grant. Luibel told them, "We need some 'walking around money.'" The AOA awarded $30,000, though at first TCOM officials only took $5,000, thinking to keep the remainder as credit. When the suggestion arose that they didn't need the money very badly if they didn't take it all, they took the balance and deposited it in a bank in Fort Worth.

The grant funding from the AOA was awarded in 1967; at the 1968 annual convention of TOMA in Houston, the college made its first serious fund-raising effort; individual physicians pledged over $100,000 for the support of the college, a response from eighty-five

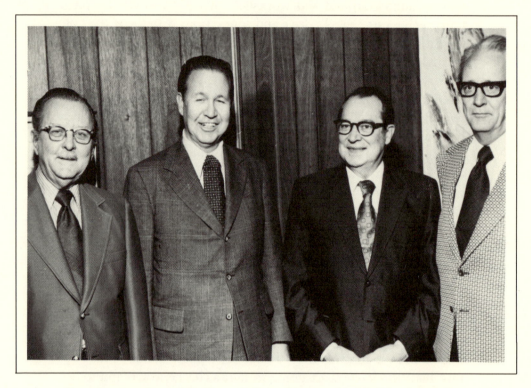

Executive committee of the Texas College of Osteopathic Medicine board of directors included, from left: Dan D. Beyer, vice-chairman; John Burnett, chairman of house and grounds; George J. Luibel, board chairman; and Carl E. Everett, secretary-treasurer. The year is 1972.

per cent of the osteopathic physicians then practicing in Texas. The state association itself authorized up to $20,000 as a grant-in-aid for the 1969-1970 fiscal year. Enthusiasm ran high.

By 1969, the college's directors realized they could not put together an operating institution on Wednesday and Thursday afternoons and weekends, the time they had free from their own professional practices. They interviewed—and hired—a native Texan with a background in public relations and some experience in fund raising. The TCOM board agreed to see if C. Ray Stokes "lives up to his clippings"; on April 15, 1969, he became the first employee of the college, with the title of Director of Development.

Stokes' first office was the den in his home. Within weeks of his hiring, he attended his first state osteopathic convention and set up a booth, "learned my way around the hospital," traveled across the state to meet various osteopathic physicians who supported the college effort, and, finally, attended an AOA convention in Chicago, visiting other osteopathic colleges on his way to and from that convention. It was a crash course in osteopathic medicine.

Stokes also hired his first employee—his wife, Edna who worked as a secretary for $1.75 an hour. She became secretary, bookkeeper and cleaning lady. "They gave me a brown envelope," Edna Stokes recalls. "It had some cancelled checks and a checkbook, and they told me that was it. I was to go ahead and set up some books."

On May 1, 1969, Stokes rented the college's first official space—a small office at 1500 West Fifth, which was rented furnished for $110 a month—and he bought the college's first equipment, an Underwood typewriter which he is still using twenty years later. Stokes bought the typewriter for sixty dollars and reported once that when he took it to be cleaned the machine was appraised as an antique and valued at fifteen hundred dollars; he didn't sell it.

Stokes was asked to prepare a statement of goals to be presented at the 1969 annual convention of TOMA in Dallas. He had only two weeks to learn all he could about osteopathic medicine—he was given a reading list—but he managed to have ready for distribution in printed form the following statement:

GOALS

—To provide a four-year postgraduate course in medical education, leading to the granting of the D.O. degree;

—To graduate sixty-four physicians annually, commencing in 1974;

—To conduct research in basic science and clinical applications of the osteopathic concepts of medicine;

—To provide health services to the community through the college hospital and clinics;

—To provide training for personnel in the allied health professions;

—To provide opportunity for postdoctoral and continuing education for practicing physicians and allied health professions personnel.

One of Stokes' early assignments was difficult and met with failure. When the effort was made to entice the Des Moines college to Fort Worth, a prominent local family had seemed interested in giving sixty acres of land northwest of the city to the college. Stokes was asked to try to revive that interest. He was unsuccessful, and the land now houses a portion of the northwest campus of Tarrant County Junior College.

But he was much more successful on his next assignment. Luibel said to him, "Hire us a dean." Faced with this challenge, Stokes, an alumnus of Texas Christian University, consulted Dean Jerome Moore at that institution, who said, "If you can get him, hire Henry Hardt."

Dr. Henry B. Hardt, a Columbia University Ph.D., began his duties as associate dean and chief administrative officer on October 1, 1969. He had retired as a chemistry professor at TCU and was working on a yearly contract as a chemistry professor at Jarvis College in East Texas. Hardt was agreeable to joining TCOM when his current obligations to Jarvis College were fulfilled. He later described himself as ideally suited to helping establish a medical school, having "a tough body and brain that was slow and stubborn, which required all the help available for such a service to

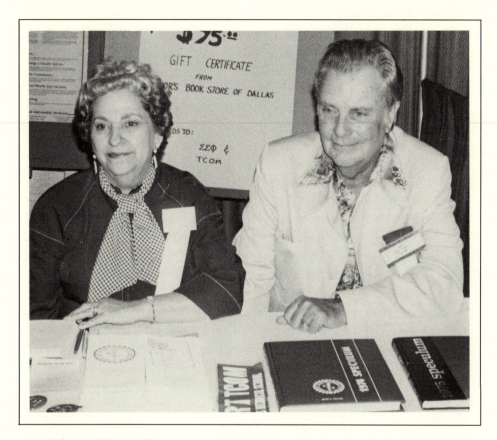

Edna and Ray Stokes, 1976.

humanity." In truth, he was a gold mine for the college. Hardt was founding president of the Texas State Board of Examiners for the Basic Sciences and served twenty years on that board, having been appointed for six-year terms by each of four governors, and he had been chairman of the department of chemistry at TCU and a member of the pre-med advisory committee. He had also twice been president of the National Collegiate Athletic Assocation and had a long list of other academic honors and associations. He was a man of dignity, comfortable in the academic world. Later, Dr. Hardt would suggest that "an absolute requirement in every good medical school instructor . . . is personal integrity, because without personal integrity, nothing else matters." Dr. Hardt was well qualified to lead the fledgling school.

As those involved with the opening of the school recall the events of 1970, Hardt's importance looms large, and his praises are sung over and over again. Says faculty member Elizabeth Harris, "He was the wisest man I have ever known. Sure, he had feet of clay—he was the most hard-headed, stubborn German!—but he had a dignity and a grace that inspired us all."

In February 1970 the college moved its offices from 1500 West Fifth Street, a good distance from FWOH, to a small house at 3600 Mattison, across the street from the hospital. The house was used for offices by Stokes, his wife, and Dean Hardt. Mrs. Stokes thinks she is the only secretary who had to clean a bathtub, but since the office was in a converted residence, there was indeed a bathtub. And there was no maid service. The budget was so tight, she remembers, that she brought a coffeepot and a pencil sharpener from home— and she used to bring the pencils too.

That spring, the 1970 TOMA convention was in Lubbock. The board of directors and college administration went to the convention to make their first "hard and fast pitch" for real money, not just pledges. It would unfortunately prove true that only $74,000 of the $100,000 pledged at the earlier convention was ever collected.

There were, of course, TOMA members who thought the college would never work, people who thought the planners knew nothing about running a college, even people who thought they could run it better.

"One doctor," says Luibel, "suggested we didn't know any more about running a college than we did about running a filling station. I told him we really didn't know anything about a filling station either. If we bought one, we'd hire a guy who knew how to run it, and we didn't expect to run a college. And we never did run the college. We always brought in people. . . ."

Luibel himself had more background for institutional planning than most practicing physicians. He had sat on the boards of both the AOA and TOMA for many years and as a member of the alumni board of the Kirksville College of Osteopathic Medicine, he had met frequently with that college's board of trustees and was therefore familiar with the workings of institutions. Later, one of his colleagues would praise Luibel not only for his faith but also for his political savvy. Another said of him, "his host of friends and some adversaries agree that he takes no neutral position on medicine, politics, economics or social implications."

And the college was doubly blessed by the presence of Hardt who, having been in the academic world, knew how to go about recruiting faculty and students. He had academic prestige, and he knew where to acquire people with doctorate degrees to teach the various basic science subjects. Those who worked with Hardt in the early days of the college have nothing but the highest praise for his professionalism, his integrity, his enthusiasm—and his determination to put the college on the right track.

In the spring of 1970, Luibel suggested to Everett that as treasurer he should make a concerted effort to raise money not only from the Texas profession but from osteopathic physicians across the country. Everett wrote two letters to every member of the AOA and got good results, close to $50,000 in cash. Everett also initiated what he called the "$1,000 Club" of people who had donated that amount to the college. One day in the spring of 1970, he invited the staff of FWOH to lunch at a local country club; before the lunch was over, he had raised $20,000 for the college. Everett emphasizes that

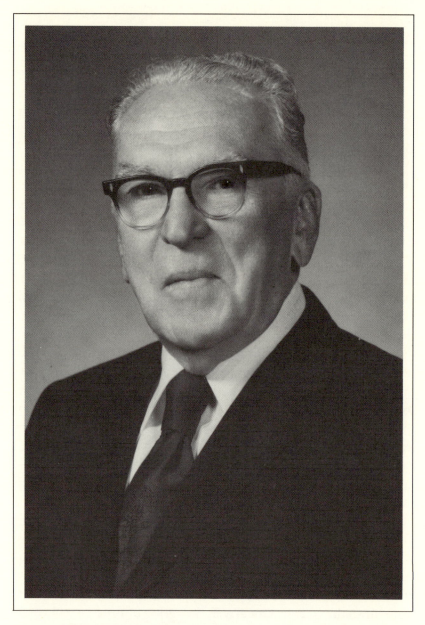

Dean and Chief Executive Officer Henry E. Hardt. The photograph was made shortly before his retirement in 1974.

support from the local osteopathic profession was extremely strong.

Hardt began quiet plans for the eventual opening of the school. The first faculty member recommended to the board of directors was Dr. Elizabeth Harris. She joined Hardt and the Stokeses in the offices in the small house by March 1970. Harris was completing doctoral work in microbiology at Southwestern Medical School. When she received a letter from Hardt, outlining the challenges at the proposed school, she was immediately interested. She left an initial meeting excited about the possibilities of teaching in a medical school.

Hardt also faced the problem of student recruitment. How does a brand new medical college recruit students? How does it put out the word that it may be ready for students in the fall? In Hardt's words, "our job consisted largely of selecting twenty newly surprised students to face a newly assembled faculty with an untried curriculum." It was, he concluded, a "near-miraculous" performance.

Little attempt was made to solicit students. Harris recalls that it was Luibel's view that if there should not be adequate funding or if something else unforeseen happened, they would not be in the embarrassing position of having solicited students only to have to tell them, "Well, sorry, we're not really going to open." Hardt did write to some propsective students, but mostly word-of-mouth, mainly in physicians' offices and by pharmaceutical representatives, was relied on to pass the news of the available freshman seats at the college. Applicants would have to understand the uncertain conditions of their enrollment including the possibility that the school might close at the end of the first year. Should that dark possibility become reality, every effort would be made to guarantee students seats at other osteopathic colleges across the country; for many, the difference in financing might have made continuation of their education impossible. Like the brand new faculty, the students entering TCOM's first class were risk-takers; perhaps, too, they were dreamers. Applications were received as early as February, although no opening date for the college had been announced.

Sometimes mistakes turn into good fortune. Through a misun-

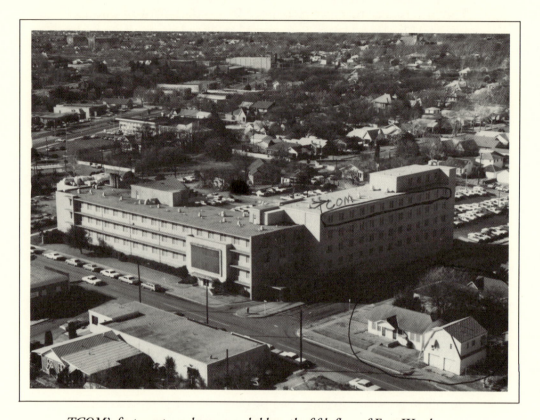

TCOM's first campus: classes were held on the fifth floor of Fort Worth Osteopathic Hospital on Montgomery Street; administrative offices were in the small white house at the lower right of this photo; the garage apartment to the far right served as the anatomy lab.

derstanding, in June the press received and publicized word that the college would open in the fall of 1970. "We didn't intend to open that soon," says Luibel, "but they blew our cover." Belatedly, the board officially announced the fall opening.

Hardt had wanted a year of planning and, according to Harris, had penned a letter to the three founders advising against the announced opening. He kept the letter in his desk drawer and was determined to send it if AOA approval was not forthcoming. The letter was never sent, and as far as Harris knows, she is the only other person who saw it.

By that time, most faculty were in place and most student applicants had been interviewed. But the college had no classroom space. Several places were investigated, but finally someone suggested the fifth floor of the hospital, then an unused shell. The idea was not viewed favorably by the board of the hospital.

Luibel was president of that board, but Russell, the physician who had secured the land for the Fort Worth Osteopathic Hospital and who was an acknowledged leader in the profession in Texas, was chairman of the FWOH board. Russell was opposed to opening the college in hospital quarters—he wanted a private hospital, not a teaching institution, and he wanted a college on more solid financial footing before it was a reality. It was a truism that as Russell went, so went the board. If he could be convinced to favor the plan, there would be no problem.

Everett volunteered to go to Russell and try to convince him. He went to the older physician's home on a Sunday. "That afternoon," remembers Everett, "we'd had a norther come in. It was very cold, and the wind was extremely high. We sat in the front room, and it was cold in there. Dr. Phil apologized for the cold, but we sat in that room for five hours."

Everett presented the board's reasons for wanting to open in the hospital, and finally, Russell said, "Well, if that's what you want to do, I'll be for it." From that moment on, says Everett, it was Russell's idea to put the college on the fifth floor of the hosital. But Fisher insists that Everett is solely responsible for the ongoing cooperation between the hospital and the college.

It was a busy summer and fall. Official approval, in the form of pre-accreditation status, did not come from the AOA until July 9, 1970. That gave Hardt less than three months to make final preparations, including finishing the classroom space on the fifth floor. October 1—later than traditional school openings—had been announced as the first day of classes in order to give the administration more time to assemble a faculty and prepare for the entrance of the first class.

Ray Stokes knows as much as anyone about the preparation of the hospital's fifth floor for opening day. "We put up partitions to divide the library, a large classroom, and a large lab. Some faculty members had offices on the fifth floor, though the college offices were still in the little white house across the street." The anatomy lab was in a garage apartment behind the house, with five cadavers for dissection. "It wasn't," says Everett, "an impressive way to start a college, but it served the purpose."

The Federal Surplus Agency provided chairs, desks, tables and more at a token cost. The greatest gift, without doubt, came from Texas Christian University which provided, free of charge, practically all the equipment and bench furniture used in the science laboratories in the fifth-floor quarters. It was a gift worth many thousands of dollars to the college.

Hardt, meanwhile, continued to recruit faculty, with what he called "the audacity to offer positions in an institution that did not exist—and might never! We stated that fact frankly and emphatically—and no one ever refused to accept the challenge." Dr. Tom Graham, a physiologist, and Dr. Charles Rudolph, a biochemist, were the next faculty members hired after Elizabeth Harris. Rudolph's wife, Diana, who held a M.S. in chemistry, became an assistant to the faculty.

Mary Lu Schunder inquired about a faculty position after reading about the college in the newspaper and was hired as the college's anatomist. Along with general surgeon Dr. George Pease, she was made a member of the Anatomical Board of the State of Texas so that the college could obtain the cadavers necessary for the gross anatomy class at the college. Schunder later joked that the size of the first class—twenty students—was in large part determined by the number of tables that would fit into the garage apartment-anatomy laboratory. Five was the maximum; at four students per table, that meant twenty students. "There were other considerations, of course," she says, "but that was an important one." In truth, the AOA had approved the college for "not more than twenty students."

The remaining members of the initial full-time faculty were Drs. Jack Banister (microbiology and biochemistry), George H. Jurek (anatomy), Joel Alter (surgery-anatomy), as well as Joan Swaim (librarian). With the addition of Diana Rudolph and Dean Hardt himself, the faculty met the minimum requirement that a medical school faculty must initially consist of at least ten members.

In looking back on those days, Harris says, "a group of people were brought together, each of whom brought his own talent, his own educational experiences, his philosophy, his commitment to the establishment of the institution . . . and it was the dedication of many of these people that allowed the college to become a reality."

A catalog was urgently needed. Hardt appointed Harris chair of the curriculum committee, with physicians Gerald Bennett and John Kemplin the other members. Hardt, Harris recalls, had a way of flattering people into helping. "We are in need of your wisdom and years of experience," he would write. The committee met at the hospital, at the suggestion of Dr. Bennett, and pored over the AOA requirements which specified 1200 clock-hours of instruction during a student's first year. In the first catalog, the courses are listed by clock-hours—273 for gross anatomy, 126 for microanatomy, 90 for neuroanatomy, and on down the list of courses for a total of 1198.

That first catalog had a white cover with red ink. That, says Harris, was because physiologist Tom Graham was assigned the job of putting the catalog together. He'd attended the University of Alabama and used his alma mater's colors, even though Hardt, Schunder and Harris all wanted purple and white, the colors of Texas Christian University in Fort Worth. In the late seventies, the white paper stock was changed for beige, and then a new director of news and information protested that the use of blood-red as a color was unfortunate for a medical school. Burgundy was substi-

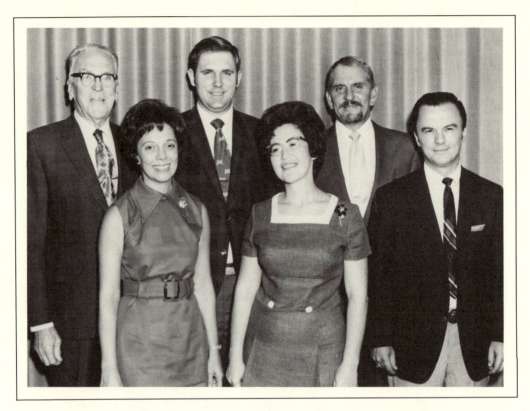

The original basic sciences faculty with Dean Hardt: Mary Lu Schunder, Elizabeth Harris and Tom Graham stand in front; Hardt, Charles Rudolph and Jack Banister are in the back.

tuted for red, and the school's colors evolved to the current burgundy and gray.

Letterhead presented similar problems of uniformity. At one
point, the college purchased stationery with the osteopathic seal in
orange, the college's name in black. Several faculty members re-
belled and purchased their own letterhead at their own expense. It
was, Harris says, very plain and simple, very "academic."

By October 1, 1970, the college was ready to embark on its great
adventure. Provisional accreditation status was granted by the AOA
the day the college officially opened.

৪৪ৠ৪ *The First Year*

Teachers everywhere confirm the belief that individual classes take on individual characteristics—some quick, some difficult, some friendly, some hostile. The Class of 1974 at TCOM was special—in many ways—and it most definitely took on a cohesiveness that blended nineteen young men and one woman into a group with a clear identity.

"The thing that sticks in my mind about that first year," says Dr. David Ray, a member of the initial class, " is that we became very close—not only the students, but the wives and the children. It was because of the stress we were under—with stress, folks tend to plunk together whenever they can for support. We were concerned about the school, concerned about our own education, concerned about doing passing work."

Dr. Elizabeth Harris remembers the group as special because of the "wonderful student/teacher interaction. . . . It was a unique and very special opportunity to teach such a small group of students." More than that, she credits the first class with outstanding motivation. "They felt as though they had suddenly been given a very special opportunity to become physicians—something that each wanted to do but for some reason or another had not had the opportunity to do until TCOM was founded."

They were also willing workers. When the class arrived for registration in late September 1970, the donated chairs and tables from TCU and the Federal Surplus Agency were stacked behind the white house that held college offices. Students and faculty pitched in to carry them to the fifth floor of the hospital. "They were twenty-four hour students," recalls Dr. Mary Lu Schunder. "They literally helped build the college."

Students and faculty were put to work in many ways that autumn. "Before we started teaching," said one faculty member, "we kept old working clothes at the office so we could change our appearance to meet the need." Dr. Jack Banister who taught microbiology and physiology joined Dean Henry Hardt in refinishing the government surplus desks for faculty use, and he enlisted the help of students and their wives to fix up the lounge area. They spent a solid week of hard work, painting and decorating.

Harris remembers that her husband, Joe, was always available to haul tables or chairs in his pickup and that Dr. Charles Rudolph, the first biochemist, installed the library shelves because "it just had to be done." Rudolph used to joke that for two months he was mistaken for a general contractor instead of a professor.

In spite of all this volunteer help, the school the first class attended was small and makeshift at best. The hospital quarters began with a large reception area. There were three faculty offices, a small office area for the "Girl Friday" (who was Rudolph's wife Diana), and a classroom, a library, a large laboratory and a student lounge. Donated items were everywhere: Vyra Everett, Carl's wife, did the paintings which hung in the reception area, a faculty member donated "early attic" furniture for the ladies lounge—the students called it "Nelda's lounge," in recognition of Nelda Cunniff, the lone female student in the first class.

The laboratory was not walled off into separate spaces for each subject, but there were areas for microscopy and biochemistry, and a section for osteopathic medicine complete with McManis treatment tables. "There was no conflict in the fact that the laboratories were all in one space," explains Harris, "because there were only twenty students, and they were all always doing the same thing at the same time."

Students and faculty alike referred to the classroom as "The Steamship" because an abuttment, designed to cover pipes, jutted into the room, giving it an odd configuration. Since the floor was flat, rather than tiered, teaching was done from a small platform. "I think it happened to everyone at least once," says Schunder. "In the heat of a lecture, you found that you fell off the edge of the platform and caught yourself on the window ledge as you went down." She also remembers that the blackboards "had been hung by someone who was six foot three, so I could only use the lower third in my lectures."

The library was approximately thirty by forty feet, with shelving on three walls. When she reported for her first day of work, librarian Joan Swaim was startled to find old metal shelving, donated by TCU, sitting in the middle of the room; on the shelves were about 4000 old medical texts. They had been shelved by Banister because he didn't want her to arrive to a library full of boxes of books. "Of course, I had to take all the books *off* the shelves and put them in the right order," Swaim says. Of the books, only about thirty were new medical texts. All had been donated.

Donations to the library came from the AOA, from TOMA, and from individual physicians. Many doctors cleaned out their offices of long-treasured medical journals and textbooks left from their own school days, thereby giving the library material of historical value. Once, a pickup truck pulled up outside the hospital, its bed loaded with somebody's garage of donations, mostly journals which Swaim had to sort. The contribution came from a physician located several hundred miles from Fort Worth.

Swaim, after touring the library facilities at John Peter Smith Hospital, Fort Worth's city-county facility, mentioned that she had not yet been able to purchase *Index Medicus,* the basic index necessary to all medical libraries; a donation followed immediately. Swaim carried the books, "a few at a time," to her fifth floor quarters.

The anatomy laboratory behind the white house was crowded but functional. David Ray still laughs over the night someone broke into the anatomy lab. "It was interesting to note that nothing was stolen. One of the body bags was opened, and that apparently was the end of the robbery. . . . They checked out of the building rather quickly after that."

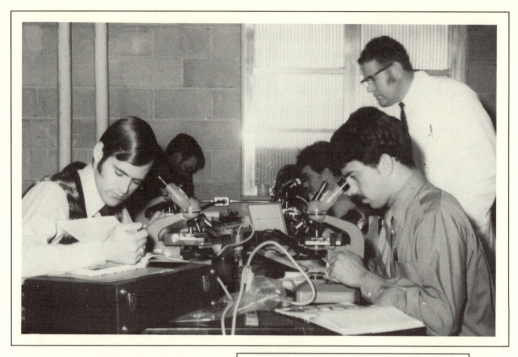

Members of the class of '74 work in the TCOM lab on the fifth floor of FWOH. At right, Joan Swaim, librarian.

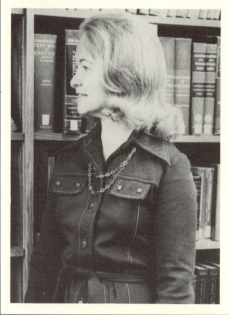

The school's one skeleton often provided a few laughs. Students dressed it in a laboratory coat and hat, put a cigarette in its mouth, and moved it as needed.

Teaching methods and materials had to be improvised constantly, and the quality of the education was a tribute to the inventiveness of the faculty and students. In clinical biochemistry and immunology, students used their own blood and urine for laboratory tests. Banister used his wife's oven at home to sterilize glassware for microbiology, and her pressure cooker became a miniature autoclave when he needed to prepare sterilized materials on which to grow bacterial cultures.

Faculty found themselves teaching outside their particular area of expertise and cramming to keep ahead of the classes. Once, recalls Dr. Virginia Ellis, "I can remember walking into Harris' office, and there she was, sitting behind her desk with old, great big fat textbooks all over the place, writing notes furiously. I said, 'Libby, what in the world are you doing?' 'Well, I've got to teach a class. . . .' I don't remember what it was, but it wasn't her field of microbiology. She said, 'We need this class taught and there isn't anybody to do it, so I'm going to.'"

Harris also wrote an early pharmacology grant proposal "by the seat of my pants, using catalogs and a whole lot of common sense to put together a logical discussion."

Basic science faculty were hired as full-time employees, but clinical faculty volunteered their time in those early basic science courses. They had their work cut out for them simply because they were unused to teaching. And, like the basic science faculty, they often taught subjects outside their area of expertise. Ellis, a pediatrician, recalls a luncheon meeting at Fort Worth Osteopathic Hospital in the winter of 1970 when a piece of paper was passed. "We were asked to consider what we would be willing to teach, and I sat next to George Luibel and whispered to him, 'I don't want to teach pediatrics.' I said if only the school were big enough, I could be dean of women. He laughed and said, 'Why don't you sign up for the history of medicine?' And I did. And that's where I started with the college—with the history of medicine. I was not a medical historian. I was not even a historian. But I tell you, it has enlarged my library, and I am fascinated by medical history."

Dr. Catherine Carlton, a longtime Fort Worth general practitioner, served as chairman of the department of osteopathic theory and technique for five years. "I didn't know how to teach. I had been in practice, but Dr. Ira Rumney of Kirksville told me what to do and sent me their books and so I started with that." She remembers being "petrified" the first time she met the freshmen students, but "they were nice young people." Eventually Carlton was asked if she wanted to go full time with the college; reluctantly, she turned the offer down in favor of private practice, but she remained a clinical associate professor of osteopathic philosophy, principles and practice.

Volunteer clinical faculty were essential to the school's early operation. Local physicians, both D.O.s and M.D.s, along with paramedical personnel, cooperated to present a full curriculum to TCOM's first class. Several courses—histology, psychology, osteopathic theory and technique, history of medicine—were taught entirely by volunteer physicians.

In addition to Carlton and Ellis, volunteer clinical faculty listed in the first catalog were Joel Alter (surgery), Raymond Beck (radiology), Edward Becka (ENT), Gerald Bennett (pathology-histology), Charles Farrow (surgery), Roy Fisher (surgery), George Grainger (osteopathic theory and technique), Constance Jenkins (physiology), William R. Jenkins (surgery), John Kemplin (radiology), George Luibel (osteopathic theory and technique), Robert Nobles (physical diagnosis), George Pease (surgery-anatomy), Phil Russell (history of medicine), Myron G. Skinner (pathlogy-histology), and Tom Whittle (medical psychology).

Grainger, a member of the board of trustees, made a 250-mile round trip once a week from Tyler, Texas, to teach osteopathic philosophy and manipulation. He closed his office, drove to Fort Worth, taught his class, and drove back to Tyler late at night. When the class studied the anatomy of a hernia, a surgeon from FWOH lectured; when the foot was studied, a podiatrist lectured; anatomy lectures on the eye were given by an ophthalmologist.

30

Stokes, as acting business manager of the college, kept a careful record of the hours donated by each volunteer faculty. He remembers that in the first year of operation, the college had eighteen doctors on its clinical science staff but none on the payroll. In February 1972, though still in the early history of the college, some clinical faculty were paid the fifty dollars an hour originally agreed upon as teaching fees. Nearly every one of them endorsed their check back to TCOM.

During its first year, the college operated primarily on funds from the osteopathic profession. Toward the end of the year, TCOM received its first federal grant of $35,000 from the U.S. Department of Health, Education and Welfare. The gift, called an institutional grant, carried no restrictions on its use. In 1971, generous grants from the J. E. and L. E. Mabee Foundation, the Amon G. Carter Foundation, and the Sid Richardson Foundation enabled the college to improve its facilities and hire additional teaching personnel.

Inevitably questions arose about the quality of education being given to students—if equipment was sometimes makeshift, and the library was scant and faculty were teaching unfamiliar subjects, were students getting a good education? David Ray remembers that students were anxious about the instruction in some classes, particularly because they failed to see continuity between teaching and lab work. "Looking back at things now, with a different perspective, some rather highly specific points don't seem so great," says Ray.

Dissatisfaction, he feels, is typical of medical students. Ray sees the conflict between the basic science emphasis in the first two years and the student's desire to work with living, breathing patients as the never-ending pressure a student puts on a medical school; the school on the other hand has certain requirements and cannot separate students by the amount of science they have had, letting some skip basic sciences and get right to clinical work. "You just have to get to the point where you have enough basic information to move on into the clinical parts of medicine." Ray's first two years in school were, he estimates, about ninety percent basic sciences, with "just enough clinical work to keep the interest up."

Ray, impressed by what he calls an "awesome act of faith" on the

31

part of the men and women who started the school, speaks of the evolutionary aspect of any educational institution. "That maybe doesn't excuse inadequacies, but it helps one keep it in perspective." Any inadequacies, he says, were overcome by the personal attention provided by the faculty and by the enormous amount of hard work done by faculty and students alike. Does he value his educational experience? "To me, just the idea of having been there that first year, the very idea of starting a medical school from scratch, from zero, it's phenomenal."

Dr. Nelda Cunniff reinforces Ray's attitude, saying, "I doubt that medical education is ever complete. I feel like I got a good basic medical education."

Schunder echoes their comments from the faculty point of view, emphasizing that the opportunity to work with students in classes of only twenty or thirty is rare. Calling it teaching "one on one," Schunder says that the close teacher-student relationship allowed faculty to spot student problems before they developed and to devote more attention to the individual student. "Our enthusiasm and our willingness to work together helped overcome most of our problems."

Later, a *Fort Worth Star-Telegram* editorial (June 2, 1974) would congratulate the first class for having endured the pain associated with being the first through a brand new medical school. "In a way, the members of the first class can look back on the college as their first 'patient,' for they presided at its birth. And the patient survived."

One caveat from the first year of the school: in recent years, the college has been referred to, by the community, as "T-COM." The faculty and staff from the days the college opened are insistent that it be known as it was then as "T-C-O-M."

The fifth floor of the hospital had always been viewed as temporary quarters. It was not, for one thing, large enough to accommodate a second class. In 1971, the college began its fall semester, with an entering class of thirty-two students, in a nearby bowling alley. One of Stokes' most embarrassing public moments came when he was misquoted as having said that TCOM was born in a bowling alley. As Stokes acknowledges, that makes a good story, but the truth is that the college was born in a hospital.

And will forever remain grateful to that hospital for its willing cooperation and its largesse during the college's struggling early years. The rent on the 10,000 square-foot fifth floor was $40,000; it was never billed to the college and never paid, although TCOM did pay monthly rent on the white house office space, also owned by the hospital, and paid utility bills for the fifth floor quarters, as well as financing the necessary heating and air conditioning equpment for the fifth floor. Luibel secured a grant of $25,000 for that purpose.

A permanent site remained an enormous problem for the college. In 1970, even before the first class entered, land in the south portion of the nearby city of Arlington had been donated by W. T. "Hooker" Vandergriff and his business associate Carlisle Cravens. Vandergriff's son, Tom, was then mayor of Arlington and a close personal friend as well as a patient of a young general practitioner in that city by the name of Bobby Gene Smith.

Smith remembers that there was a lot of interest in the college when he was first in practice in the mid-sixties, but everyone felt that such a project would be an enormous amount of work. "There was kind of a thing going around then—let George do it. And, of course, George Luibel did it, because he's the kind of person who knew who to call on to make it all come together."

Smith, elected president of TOMA in 1970, became a college supporter. When the location of the college seemed a problem, Smith turned to his friend and patient. Vandergriff's father and Cravens owned fifty acres and were interested in donating it with some restrictions on the use of the land. Immediately there was controversy.

"There were those who thought, 'This is great—don't let the sun set until we get that signed over to us.' Then there were others who said, 'no,'" Smith recalls. "They said, 'That's just an unplowed cornfield out there, and we don't want that sort of thing.'" Smith arranged a meeting in February 1970 between Tom Vandegriff and the board of the college, because he did not want to solicit the gift of land only to have it rejected by the college. The land was accepted, and the college had a home, at least a temporary one.

Stokes sees the gift as the deciding factor that influenced the AOA Board of Trustees to give pre-accreditation status to the college on July 9, 1970. On paper the property boosted the college's assets some $300,000—enough to give the "paper college" a certain financial stability. But Luibel calls the gift one that he always had "mixed emotions" about.

"The gift had a clause that if we ever ceased to use the land for educational purposes, it would revert to them and their heirs. Now I can understand they weren't going to give it to us and let us turn around and sell it in a few years, but if they had said at the end of twenty years or so, we would obtain clear title, I would have felt better about it. . . . Otherwise, no matter what investment we put on it, if it turned out that this was not right for us, that we couldn't, for reason of facilities or hospital connections or anything else, or community support, or a myriad of other reasons, or inaccessiblity for the rest of the profession, we couldn't afford to be in a position where we had money tied up in buildings or equipment that were difficult to move."

At the time, the south Arlington location was remote and isolated. It is now adjacent to a major highway and has easy access from both Dallas and Fort Worth—a point Smith had long touted in its favor—but in 1970 no one could foresee urban sprawl and the direction it would take. Ultimately, the land was returned to the donors.

Luibel insists he always felt that the college should be in Fort Worth, because it was the only major Texas city without a professional school. Looking ahead to the next hurdle for TCOM, he remarks, "We could get more legislative support for something like this than if we tried to put it in Dallas, Houston or San Antonio."

The problem of a permanent site remained. In seeking both rental and permanent property, Stokes toured a variety of sites—a former Corps of Engineers Building, a warehouse on Jacksboro Highway, the Fort Worth Christian School. The Fort Worth Independent School District had a building near downtown Fort

Worth, but it was too small; the old Laneri High School was available, but only to a project related to the Catholic Church. The First Baptist Church was for sale, but the price was two million dollars, and the college was only willing to go one million; a contract was almost signed on the old Texas and Pacific passenger depot, for the tenth and eleventh floors, but it fell through. At one point, the college almost acquired what was known as the old Narcotics Farm—there was a tentative two-year agreement, negotiated by U.S. Representative Jim Wright, for the college to use the federal property; federal regulations required that it be offered first to federal agencies, and, as Stokes says, "the correctional people wanted it." It is now the Fort Worth Federal Correctional Institute, sixty acres in the southeast section of the city. The list of possible sites—none of them just right—seemed endless.

The college's next temporary quarters were not perfect either, but the location and building had several advantages. The former Tavener Bowling Alley, located at 3516 Camp Bowie Boulevard, just a block from the hospital, became the TCOM Basic Science Building and added 16,000 square feet to the college's facilities, housing classrooms, laboratories for anatomy, biochemistry, and pharmacology, along with most administration and faculty offices and the student lounge. By 1973, with the five basic science departments moved to Denton, the building would be formally called the Administration Building but forever known as "the bowling alley."

In September 1971, a first-year class of eighteen and a second-year class of thirty-two regular and two special students began study in the bowling alley. Physical facilities had been enlarged; the curriculum had been expanded; additional faculty had been added.

Proof of success came in the spring of 1972 when the first class was examined by the National Board of Examiners in Osteopathic Medicine and Surgery. TCOM students scored higher than students from four of the other seven osteopathic colleges in all categories but one. The college was off and running.

﷯ *State Affiliation: The Road to Denton*

T HE FIRST STATE AID TO TCOM CAME WITH THE PASSAGE AND subsequent signing by Governor Preston Smith on May 17, 1971, of Senate Bill 160. This enabling legislation allowed the Coordinating Board, Texas College and University System, to contract with TCOM to provide for the education of *bona fide* Texas resident undergraduate medical students pursuing the degree of Doctor of Osteopathy.

The state osteopathic association—TOMA—had been receiving some scholarship funds to assist students pursuing a career in osteopathic medicine out of state because there was no college in Texas. That came about because several years earlier a politically active osteopathic physician, Dr. Elmer Baum of Austin, found that the state was assisting students who were studying forestry out of state because no comparable curriculum was offered in Texas. Baum said, in effect, "Hey, here's another group who are pursuing an education out of state. How about giving us some funding for this?" Scholarships began with token amounts but gradually worked up to a point where the association was given $100,000 annually. In the early sixties, that project had occupied much of the time of the TOMA committee appointed to study the feasibility of an osteopathic college in Texas.

The state association also learned that Baylor University was receiving funds to assist in providing medical education. The two situations, according to Bobby Gene Smith, were used to map out a direction for TCOM in pursuing funding from the state.

TCOM had asked for help from the state association in seeking this funding, and because Smith was then president the responsibilty fell on his shoulders. It was complicated, he says, when news came that the TOMA lobbyist at that time might possibly be involved in a bank scandal. The lobbyist offered to step aside until the matter was cleared, but that left no one to present the case in Austin, except Smith and the association's executive director, Tex Roberts. Roberts, who had only recently moved from a similar position in New Mexico, was deeply committed to the college's future and an able ally for Smith.

"I had never involved myself in anything like that," says Smith. "I hardly knew my senator, and that was it. I guess maybe part of the reason for my success was that I didn't know you couldn't do it."

Smith was told that the way to start was to get his senator to sponsor a bill. Because of gerrymandering, the Arlington physician's senator was Tom Creighton from Weatherford. Creighton proved more than helpful. "Time and time again," remembers Smith, "he'd call and say 'You'd better get down here because this is what's happening,' so Tex Roberts and I would jump on a plane or get in a car and buzz off down there and do whatever he said to do. It was a day-to-day sort of thing, with no real plan for tomorrow because you didn't know what tomorrow would bring."

One tomorrow brought real concern from a Galveston senator, a senior member of the state senate with key assignments. A. R. "Babe" Schwartz "asked pointed questions," Smith says, "and it soon became apparent we had a real problem." Schwartz's major concern was that he wanted the state auditor to oversee any allocated funds. "He didn't want to give the money to a bunch of doctors and have them go to Las Vegas to spend it," explains Smith, "and I could understand that." Senator Creighton recommended that Smith and Roberts present themselves at Schwartz's office early one morning to resolve the matter.

They did. "We're here to try to deal with your concerns about our bill," Smith told him. "What is it that you don't like?" So they talked . . . and talked . . . and Schwartz told them it was their bill and he wouldn't change it, but he made certain recommendations. Smith sums it up by saying that they wanted the same things Schwartz did—state auditing of the funds—but that they hadn't known to write it into the bill. "It was a good thing," Smith insists, "for the profession to be answerable to the state."

In the end, the association sacrificed the out-of-state funding, putting that money into the TCOM bill. The state added another $50,000, and the college was funded for $150,000 for one year. "We had something to pay our teachers," Smith says, "and it was a great feeling. . . ." TCOM—operating on a shoestring—got its foot in the state's door.

The bill was signed May 17, 1971, five months after Smith and Roberts had first become lobbyists. At a celebration in his office, Creighton told Smith, "The only reason you ever got this bill passed is because nobody told you you couldn't." Smith believed him.

The next year, the governor revoked the entire second half of the biennial budget and went back to the legislature to create a new budget for the second biennium. By then the college had operated successfully for a year on the $150,000 and administrators had demonstrated that they could spend their money wisely. Their allocation was doubled for the next biennium.

That amounted to about $12,000 per *bona fide* Texas student. "It enabled us to use some of our other monies to consolidate our position," says Luibel. "We paid off some debts and bought some property around us." Soon the college's assets amounted to three million dollars—a fact that would be of major importance when they sought affiliation with a state university.

"Some schools come into a state with that much in assets, but it's vacant land—a farm or something—on the edge of town. We were a medical school in the middle of town—where a medical school needs to be to function effectively—with three million dollars worth of assets. There were buildings, usable buldings, on our land," Luibel explains.

By 1972 the college owned a square block near the Fort Worth

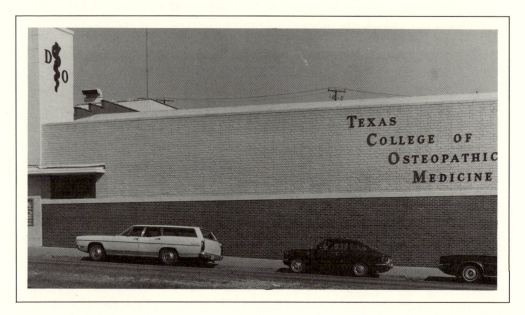

The Bowling Alley.

Osteopathic Hospital, plus a nearby lot and building. The property contained, in the words of Luibel, "a bowling alley, a motel, a 'go-go' joint, and a liquor store. . . . We should have kept the liquor store in business until we became a state school."

The next building purchased was a small structure originally built in 1926 as a laundry and fur storage facility. By the time the college bought it, it was a used furniture store and in poor repair, although the outside walls and beams were sound. It was acquired with a grant from the J. E. and L. E. Mabee Foundation and remodelled and enlarged with aid from the United States Department of Health, Education and Welfare. The government grant was called "start-up money" and was designated for hiring faculty.

Finding teachers proved difficult, however, and college officials were frustrated that the grant money was there but could not be used where it was most needed. Eventually approval was secured from Washington to use the money for remodeling rather than for hiring faculty. In spite of rumors that the college was in bad trouble for misuse of HEW funds, the remodeling proceeded smoothly. The same source of money later helped the college improve the top floor of the biology building on the campus of NTSU.

The bowling alley was the most recognizable structure, and TCOM's central administrative and classroom building was known simply as "the bowling alley." If anyone suggested a lack of dignity in this, Luibel reminded them that Southwestern Medical School in Dallas had begun in an old army barracks.

But, like the fifth floor of the hospital, the bowling alley needed work. When the school first occupied the building, college officials had two weeks to convert it into a school. A general surgeon bought thirty gallons of paint and joined a couple of other faculty members and some students in spending a weekend painting, changing bowling lanes into laboratories, creating administrative offices, a lobby, a library and two classrooms.

The college rented the bowling alley the first year with the aid of a grant from Fort Worth's Carter Foundation, but in the second year they signed a contract to turn rental payments into lease-to-purchase payments.

"We had a party," recalls Luibel. "The state association met in Fort Worth in 1972, and we brought them all out to the bowling alley in buses. They were amazed at how much space we had, what a good facility. So the hue and cry about location pretty much settled down." At that point, the Arlington land was returned to its owners, with grateful thanks.

The college took another giant step in 1972—it hired its first president. Marion E. Coy, a general practitioner from Jackson, Tennessee, was attending a board meeting of the AOA when Luibel, also a board member, asked him if he'd like to have a place in the administration of TCOM. Coy visited the school in January 1972 and was later told that the job was his if he wanted it. His decision to give up private practice after many years was complicated by his job that year as president of the AOA, a position that required a great deal of travel.

"But the college needed someone to get started," Coy says, so it was agreed that he would use Fort Worth, instead of Jackson, Tennessee, as his home base between trips. He completed his term as AOA president in July 1972 and from then on devoted his full attention to the growing school.

Coy saw that his biggest and most immediate challenge was to unite the osteopathic profession in Texas behind the school. By then, the institution had an unfortunate history of rumors and half truths. With Dr. Clifford Dickey, a Fort Worth general practitioner, Coy organized "Friends of TCOM" and began to invite the profession to dinner parties featuring frank discussions of progress at TCOM. The purpose was to tell the college's story throughout the state. "We tried to let them know that we were conducting this thing the way they would want an osteopathic medical school to be conducted, the way it would have to be to be accredited by the AOA and the Texas Board of Medical Examiners. . . . Some of their concerns just reflected that they didn't understand the situation. One thing I heard was 'The college isn't even accredited by their own state board of examiners.' They didn't realize that no school could be accredited until it graduated its first class."

Coy remembers spending a lot of time "trying to straighten

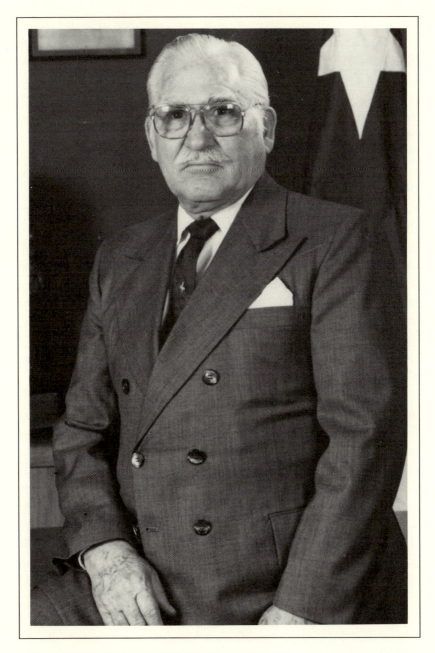

Marion E. Coy, D.O., president from 1973 to 1975.

things out" and Luibel suggests that anyone trying to found or run a medical school must learn to deal with rumors. Stokes recalls that Hardt once got a letter from a physician in Dallas who said he would like to teach at the college but he understood that only local physicians were put on the faculty and he had no chance. Dr. Hardt invited the physician to visit the college and learn about it instead of listening to rumors.

Years later, Bobby Smith recalled the period of divisiveness over the college and said the signing of Senate Bill 160 was "the greatest thing for the osteopathic profession in Texas. . . . It gave us a financial base and a way to train our kind of physicians, but greater than that it brought us together. . . ."

With a full-time educational administration, an operating campus, and assets on its balance sheet, the college sought affiation with a state institution. Luibel had never forgotten the advice of the state officer who'd told him to start the school first and then seek state affiliation. By 1972 it was time.

"Building a new medical college is a project so tremendous that union with an established academic educational institution is an almost definite requirement," says Stokes.

"We were growing," says Everett, "we were admitting classes, and it was time that we had to make progress. We had to have more faculty, more teaching equipment. There is just no end to what we needed to make a first-class medical school. But we were not a school endowed with any money."

Preliminary investigations actually began in 1971, before Coy took over as president. In November of that year, a committee of the Texas coordinating board for higher education came to look over the young school before the board would agree to recognize it. At first, recalls Luibel, they were going to gather experts from across the country. "It would have slowed us way down, and there would have been more experts than there were students and faculty put together." Eventually, two men came, one the director of medical education for the American Medical Association in Chicago and the other Dr. G. V. Brindley of Temple, Texas, a member of the coordinating board. The Chicago man, after saying he didn't think this was the right way to start a medical school, went on to say he'd have done the same thing in the same situation. Brindley said they would recommend to the coordinating board that they contract with the school but that TCOM should have some sort of an affiliation with a major university in the area. He did not specify a state school, but as the college board members did some "feeling around," they found that NTSU in Denton was more receptive than other schools. "The University of Texas at Arlington was not interested," Luibel remembers, "and the private institutions in the area—Texas Christian University and Texas Wesleyan College—were not in a financial position to take on the expense of a medical school."

Fate works in strange ways, even in the affairs of a medical school. Dr. J. K. G. Silvey, distinguished professor of biological sciences at North Texas State University in Denton, was invited to speak at the October 1971 convention of the AOA in Hawaii. Silvey was known to have a great concern for medical education, and it was said that no student he had recommended for medical school had ever been turned down. Drs. Robert Nobles and Art Wiley, osteopathic physicians practicing in Denton, had talked to Silvey and Dr. Vernon Scholes of the NTSU biology department, hoping to affect a relationship between NTSU and TCOM, but nothing formal had come out of those talks by the time of the Hawaii convention.

In Hawaii, Silvey met with Luibel and others and a question took shape in his mind: Why would a state as big and as wealthy as Texas not be able to train doctors in osteopathic medicine, so they must go some other place and then come back to Texas? Back in Denton, he called President C. C. "Jitter" Nolen.

Nolen had been inaugurated as president of the state university in August, only months before receiving Silvey's call, but he later said that the phone call fit in with what he had said in his inaugural address: "North Texas is not equipped to be all things to all persons, but it is clear we have the resources to be of more service to more persons than we are at this time."

Silvey later recalled the conversation this way: "I said, 'This is Gwynn Silvey. Would you like a medical school?' He said, 'What do

45

you mean?' I replied, 'Would you like to have a medical school as a part of North Texas?' He said, 'Why, sure.' I said, 'Are you busy?' He said, 'Not too busy.' I said, 'I'll be over to see you.'"

After Silvey and Nolen talked, both men agreed that the idea of some kind of affiliation with the new osteopathic school was worth further exploration. That December, Nolen and Dr. Gus Ferré, academic vice-president of the university, went to visit Nobles at his clinic. Nolen confesses he knew little about osteopathic medicine at the time, but Nobles talked to them and gave them reading material.

While Ferré talked to deans and department heads at NTSU to see if it was possible to offer classes on the campus to osteopathic students, Silvey began to talk to former students in medical practice—officers in the state medical association, specialists, faculty at Scott & White Memorial Hospital in Temple, Texas. They all liked the possibility. By January 1972, Ferré and Silvey were talking to NTSU faculty members, assessing their interest in the project. Some feared that the medical school would infringe on their research appropriations, but once assured there would be no such conflicts, they became supporters.

On January 11, 1972, representatives of TCOM and North Texas met in Fort Worth. They discussed what Luibel later called a "lend-lease" program whereby TCOM could "lease some of their facilities and faculty to give us some instant bricks and mortar for use in the basic science program in the first two years." Another meeting, and then a bus trip to Denton which, incidentally, occurred during Coy's initial exploration of TCOM so that he was able to join the TCOM Board of Directors on their visit.

The bus ride back to Fort Worth was lively, with a few dissenting voices, but the board of TCOM voted to accept the NTSU offer. The university proposed to teach the first year of the TCOM program on its Denton campus for $48,000 a year, or $1000 per student. It wasn't an expensive price for a medical school.

The program, which began in the fall of 1972, gave NTSU a "professional dimension that couldn't be acquired by any other means at that time," according to Nolen. "A university as large, as complex

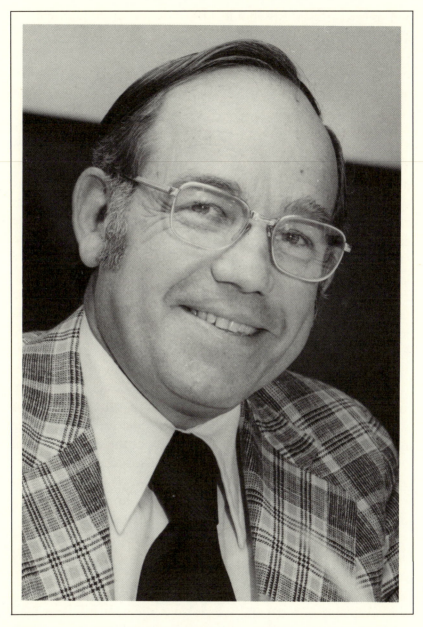

C. C. "Jitter" Nolen, who served as president of both NTSU and TCOM from 1975 to 1979. Under his leadership, TCOM made the transition to a state-supported medical school.

and as strong as NTSU should offer this service to the State of Texas."

The gross anatomy lab was located on the fourth floor of the biology building, previously an unfinished floor. When TCOM requested additional classroom space for the medical school courses, NTSU renovated a lounge area in Terrill Hall, a retired dormitory near the biology and chemistry buildings, into classroom space. The resulting classroom was long and narrow, with a lecture stand and a blackboard raised several feet so that it would be visible to students in the back of the room. "It has often been said, that keen eyesight was a necessary attribute of that first class on the NTSU campus," says Dr. Ben Harris, now associate dean for basic sciences and research and at that time NTSU coordinator of the program. (TCOM coordinator Elizabeth Harris and Ben Harris are not related.)

Eventually, in the mid-seventies, all TCOM classrooms and laboratories were located in the fourth floor of the biology building at Denton. TCOM faculty were given offices on the third floor of Terrill Hall, an area with "a paucity of air conditioners," according to Ben Harris, who adds that "midnight requisitions" from other vacant rooms on the same floor made it possible to cool the faculty offices and student study rooms. "It was rumored that these acquisitions were made by a few astute medical students, but these rumors were never verified. No one ever complained about the missing air conditioners, so one presumes that no one missed them."

Although Ben Harris was coordinator, Nolen turned academic responsiblity for the program over to Ferré, who said in retrospect that his duties were to get funding, to secure faculty, and to get full state approval for the program. "And behind all that, of course, was an adequate basic health science program. . . . We were never interested in NTSU doing the clinical years. That didn't belong to us and was not our concern. . . . But we had to get a curriculum that was acceptable to TCOM and acceptable to the standard that we had in mind, in terms of the correlation between allopathic medicine and osteopathic medicine."

For TCOM the affiliation provided additional help in the basic

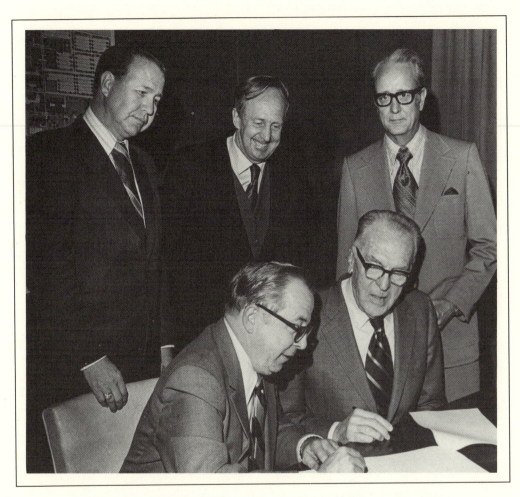

North Texas State University and Texas College of Osteopathic Medicine officials make their partnership formal: seated are A. M. Willis, chairman of the NTSU board of regents, and Henry Hardt; standing are John Burnett, TCOM, Gus Ferré, NTSU, and Carl Everett, TCOM.

sciences and a climate for research not usually emphasized in a free-standing osteopathic medical school. It also provided some additional faculty, although the first year most of the courses in anatomy, biochemistry, physiology and immunology were taught by TCOM faculty who were now employed by NTSU and who commuted to Denton, as did the students.

In the fall of 1973, the program was expanded to include some second-year courses and several new faculty were hired to teach for TCOM on the NTSU campus. In spite of its advantages, the program had its difficulties.

"It separated our student body," says Luibel. "The freshmen and sophmores really didn't meet the juniors and seniors." Coy explains, "The first year students felt like they were divorced from us. They were people without a country—graduate students in an undergraduate university. They were 'our' people, yet they were 'up there.'"

Transportation between the two schools proved difficult. TCOM basic science faculty like Schunder and Elizabeth Harris found the commute to Denton wearisome, and students wanted buses to ride back and forth. "When we had the buses," says Coy, "they'd want to come in their cars. And we couldn't economically run a thirty-five or forty-passenger bus without quite a few people in it."

Elizabeth Harris was in charge of student-related matters pertaining to the contract with NTSU—she remembers commuting to Denton and "lots of headaches. . . . It was probably two years before we even got a sign on that campus reflecting the basic sciences of TCOM—no one up there knew what TCOM was or that we were there." The program was not a separate basic health science department but functioned under the department of biology.

One further disadvantage of the split campus was that it required students to be patient about postponing their introduction to clinical experience. Ferré explains, "Most of them would like to get into the clinical experience as early as possible. And sometimes it is a good idea to do so, but since the campuses were separated it meant that they would have to postpone any clinical experience until after the basic health sciences."

Whatever difficulties the contractual arrangement with NTSU posed, it set the stage for an important and growing friendship between the private institution and the state government. For both NTSU and TCOM there was the constant thought that the program was one of exploration. Ferré says, "We would explore first for a few years, and then decide if we wanted to make a solid committment. And that would depend upon the fact that we wanted excellence. . . . We didn't hesitate to set a higher goal, and in our thinking it would be helpful to the osteopathic profession and also to the students if they had a broader curriculum than what we'd seen when we first looked at things."

The affiliation between the two schools operated for one year—1972—without state funding, but part of the agreement was that they would join in approaching the legislature for funds. In 1973, the two schools made the first successful approach to the state, securing enough *per capita* funds to pay for teaching services at NTSU.

In 1973, the former controller of North Texas, Jack Robason, was asked to serve as a liaison officer between the two schools. He began spending two to three days a week in Fort Worth, advising the then-private medical school on state requirements for operations.

By 1974, Coy was traveling the state, telling the TCOM story to the public and to legislators; and he was attending every meeting of the coordinating board. There was, simultaneously, talk of a state-supported medical school in South Texas; and Texas Women's University in Denton wanted to establish a medical school. There were nervous moments for TCOM's leaders, but ultimately the coordinating board decided there were enough allopathic medical schools in the state. Their prediction was that, with the current schools in operation *(including* TCOM), Texas would have an adequate supply of physicians in the next ten to fifteen years.

In 1975, a bill to unite the two schools—NTSU and TCOM—was introduced to the legislature, and once again osteopathic officials found themselves commuting to Austin to support legislation in their favor. Coy credits Texas Representative Gib Lewis and Senator Betty Andujar with carrying the bill through their respective

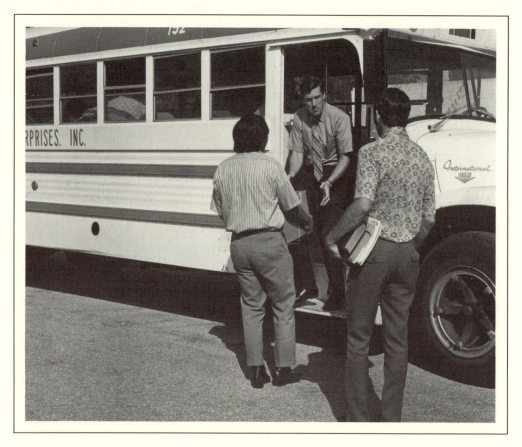

TCOM students board one of the buses that ferried them back and forth to classrooms in Denton.

legislative bodies. "About twice a week," he recalls, "I'd get a call from Dr. Andujar [the senator's husband, a practicing Fort Worth M.D.], saying he'd just got a call from her and she wanted him to call and tell me so and so. I was kept informed directly on what was going on down there."

When he introduced the bill, Representative Lewis emphasized that placing the existing, operating school in the state system would make possible its rapid expansion toward the goal of producing one hundred new physicians each year, graduates who would become family physicians. In spite of the coordinating board's predictions that Texas would have an adequate supply of physicians in ten or fifteen years, Lewis pointed out that some twenty Texas counties at that time were without one physician. Clearly, the general practitioners to be educated at TCOM were desperately needed in many areas of the state.

In May 1975 the Texas Legislature passed Senate Bill 216 which provided that TCOM become a state-supported medical school under the jurisdiction of the NTSU board of regents and president. The bill clearly specified that the school was not a school of, a college of, a branch of, or a division of NTSU. It remains a separate institution.

TCOM ended its years as a private institution with an admirable record of outside funding: Over $500,000 in federal grants, secured through strong assistance by Representative Jim Wright and Senator John Tower; nearly $400,000 from grants from private institutions—the Amon G. Carter Foundation, the Sid W. Richardson Foundation, both of Fort Worth, and the J. E. and L. E. Mabee Foundation of Tulsa, Oklahoma; an individual gift from a loyal patient of $70,000; and over $800,000 from Texas osteopathic physicians. "We fell short of the one million dollar goal from the profession," says Stokes, "but we topped that figure after we became a state school."

In August 1975, when the NTSU board of regents sat for the first time as the TCOM governing board, they met in Fort Worth. August 30 was officially designated TCOM Day in Fort Worth, and an eight-page section in the newspaper was devoted to the college. It was a day of formalities, with an academic procession and speeches by the

NTSU board chairman, president of TOMA Mike Calabrese, president of the student body Steve Farmer, alumni president David Ray, and Mayor Cliff Overcash of Fort Worth. Luibel, on behalf of the TCOM board, formally turned over some two-and-a-half milion dollars in assets, saying, "We are in the position of a gentleman giving away his only daughter to a groom he approves of." TCOM had come a long way since the days the records were kept in a brown bag.

At that time only one other state institution in the nation— Michigan State University—supported an osteopathic medical school. "That was the only available model," recalls Nolen, "and we soon learned we didn't want to do things the same way they did. Uniting the two schools under one administration posed problems that had to be worked out—NTSU faculty members worried about the new school draining resources from the university; members of the university's board of regents, not fully understanding the collaborative effort, sought information about this strange new program and too often found themselves talking only to M.D.s instead of D.O.s; Ph.D.s on the NTSU faculty objected to the salary differential between D.O.s and themselves; members of the state osteopathic association feared state control of their institution."

To deal with these and other problems, Gus Ferré was appointed interim vice president for medical affairs. He took a one-year leave of absence from his duties at NTSU to serve as chief administrative officer of TCOM. Ferré saw his mission as two-fold: to secure adequate leadershp and funding, and to request national and state monies for the construction of new buildings. Ferré visited all the existing osteopathic colleges to examine their equipment, look at their leadership, and, he hoped, learn from their mistakes. As he met with leaders of osteopathic education, Ferré noticed that one name kept surfacing: Dr. Ralph Willard of Michigan State University College of Osteopathic Medicine. It is a name that would surface again with major importance to TCOM.

As a private school, the college had necessarily run with a less formal structure than that required of state institutions. Its policies on personnel, purchasing, budget, and similar adminsitrative func-

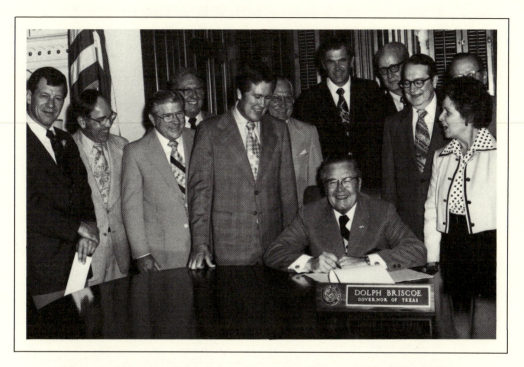

May 1975: Governor Dolph Briscoe signs Senate Bill 216. From left to right are William P. Hobby, lieutenant governor, C. C. Nolen, Claude Rainey of FWOH, Gerald P. Flanagan, D.O., Tarrant County Representative Gib Lewis, Marion Coy, Bobby Gene Smith, Carl Everett, George Luibel, Danny Beyer and Senator Betty Andujar.

tions were almost non-existent, according to L. L. LaRue, who was appointed associate dean for administration after the merger.

"My first task was to set up a budget," he recalls, "and a procedure wherein department chairman had some authority for getting out purchase orders and having things happen." Under LaRue's direction, a purchasing manual and a personnel handbook went into effect, accounting procedures were instituted. "I saw there were a lot of things to be done," he recalls, "and I rushed right into those things without spending a lot of time negotiating with those around me about how we should do it and what we should do." LaRue ruffled some feathers, but it was due to his efforts that the college expanded into the River Plaza facilities in 1977. In the late seventies, he left the campus to lobby in Austin for TOMA, returning to TCOM again in 1980.

Summing up this period in the college's history, Nolen says, "This was a huge program with a large budget and a lot of students and a program relying on medical skills and practices which occurred one hundred years ago and were being brought up to date in modern fashion. New osteopathic schools were coming into being all over the country. . . ."

Looking back at the formative years of TCOM, Nolen continues, "I think the thing that struck me was the total unselfishness. . . . The three founders so unselfishly gave the results of their work to the State of Texas and the state association joined in. . . . That makes the quality of life better and gives all of us inspiration to be better human beings than we are."

ʠʢ   *The Buildings of a Medical School*

Important as the signing of Senate Bill 216 was, it was not the college's first, nor perhaps its most important red-letter day. That day had come on June 3, 1974, when TCOM graduated its first class of eighteen physicians. "They were the first D.O.s ever to graduate from Texas," says Luibel, "and you know that was something I had heard talked about for better than twenty years around the state. This time, it happened."

In January of that year an inspection team from the Bureau of Professional Education of the AOA had recommended the college for full accreditation; a month earlier, in December 1973, an inspection team from the Texas State Board of Medical Examiners had recommended full recognition of TCOM to their board, recognition that meant that TCOM graduates would be eligible to take the state licensure examination. The college had passed two crucial tests, and the first graduation was in a sense a celebration of the school's permanency.

Henry Hardt had made it known all along that his deanship was a temporary position; he was, after all, a man well into retirement when he took over the challenge. He stayed with the college until the first class graduated in 1974, no doubt a milestone that confirmed the worth of his efforts. The college's first yearbook, the 1974 *Speculum,* is dedicated to Hardt "who led the college in its most difficult times . . . and who always put the students first."

In the fall of 1975 TCOM began its life as a state school with full accreditation, a new administration, a supportive board of regents in Denton . . . and a sprawling, second-hand campus.

Even with basic sciences classes meeting at NTSU in Denton, the Fort Worth campus was growing. It was a process of acquiring property as it became available and possible. Two outpatient clinics were opened—the first, in July 1973, was the Rosedale Clinic on the east side of the city in a predominantly low income area; the second, called Central Clinic, was a half block from the administration building, on Camp Bowie Boulevard. Housed in the former furniture store with the clinic were the pathology department, an autopsy amphitheatre, and a pathology museum. The 1974 dedication of Central Clinic on Camp Bowie proved to be quite an affair, attracting community leaders, most of the Tarrant County legislative delegation, representatives from the Tarrant County and Texas medical associations. George Luibel and U.S. Representative Jim Wright cut the ceremonial ribbon.

The school was given a Tree of Hippocrates, supposed to have been a growth from the original tree under which Hippocrates practiced medicine. It was a delicate little thing, according to then-president Coy, and "we tried to take care of it and put it into someone's hands [Kitty Bates, assistant to Ray Stokes] that we thought had a green thumb. They nursed it, but it gave up the ghost."

In 1976, the college also leased a recently vacated bank building about half a mile from the main campus. Called the Administration Building Annex, it housed the business office, admissions, the registrar's and other offices, and the department of osteopathic philosophy, principles and practice.

The winter of 1975–76 found faculty offices, the audiovisual department, public relations and alumni affairs in the Office Annex— one wing of the old motel on Camp Bowie between the bowling alley and FWOH. Plans were to raze a second wing for space for a basic science building. And in 1977, 38,000 square feet were leased in a just-completed office park, River Plaza, scenically located on the Trinity River about two miles from the Camp Bowie location. LaRue had twice proposed this arrangement to the NTSU Board of

Regents before finally acquiring approval. Acquisition of the River Plaza facility allowed the college to move the bulk of the basic science program from Denton to the new quarters on the river. The library and audiovisual department also went to River Plaza. For a while, some offices—purchasing, receiving, physical plant—were in vacant space in a large building across the street from River Plaza—coincidentally, the building also housed yet another bowling alley.

The first five years of the college were thus characterized by an extraordinary amount of moving—this office to that space, that department to this building. Clearly, it was time to build a central campus. The man who would oversee the major building program at TCOM assumed the position of dean of TCOM on November 1, 1975. He was Ralph Willard, former associate dean of the Michigan State University College of Osteopathic Medicine. Willard, a surgeon and decorated World War II Air Force veteran, was the son of two osteopathic physicians. Although Ferré stayed at TCOM for some time to oversee the transition of leadership, he eventually returned to his duties at NTSU.

Willard's appointment coincided with the announcement of the first major phase of the college's building program—and both announcements were made at the August 1975 Fort Worth meeting of the NTSU board of regents.

The first building, Medical Education Building I, was to be built with just under eight million dollars in state appropriations and over four million in construction funds from the U.S. Department of Health, Education and Welfare. Although plans all along had been to build a basic science building first, "Med Ed I" was designed to house clinical departments, the Central Clinic, an auditorium, administrative offices, the library and a few research laboratories, because federal funding could be obtained for the specific purpose of building clinics. Ground was broken for the new building by Texas Governor Dolph Briscoe on the 16th of November, 1976—a cold, rainy day brightened by the excitement over new quarters for the school.

Willard had appointed Ken Coffelt, director of biomedical communication, as his assistant, and he told Coffelt, "I want you to bird-dog the construction of Med Ed I." Coffelt was to sit in on meetings, work with planning directors at NTSU, and keep Willard informed of progress.

Coffelt recalls that Med Ed I was one of the first large precast concrete buildings to go up in the Dallas-Fort Worth metroplex. The concrete parts were poured elsewhere, trucked in, and "put together like a giant erector set." Coffelt still believes that one reason the building was completed a whopping eighteen months ahead of schedule is that it was built of precast parts.

"One of the things that stands out in my memory," says Coffelt, "is the lifting of one of the largest pieces that went into Med Ed I, the great big piece right at the top of the south end. . . . It took two big cranes to lift it, and everybody at the school turned out to witness it. We were all standing around looking and everyone holding their breath."

The other factor behind the early completion of the building was the contractor, Rooney and Associates of Florida. Coffelt says, "Mike Miller was the building superintendent for the company, and he really did an excellent job." Coffelt also credits LaRue: "He brought with him a tremendous amount of state experience. . . . He knew how to use the system."

Staging of construction on Med Ed I was critical because TCOM had to continue to operate as a school, and the new building sat nearly on top of the bowling alley, then used as college headquarters and classrooms. "When we moved into Med Ed I," says Coffelt, "the move had to be done almost overnight. We had to shut down on a Friday and open up again on Monday. We tried moving everything over a weekend—we weren't successful, but we got close." Med Ed I was occupied in August 1978. Within days TCOM faculty, staff and students were treated to the sight of bulldozers wrecking the bowling alley to make way for a parking lot. It was a moment of mixed joy and nostalgia; at least 150 of the bricks from the bowling alley were saved, cleaned, and made into mementos.

There was uncertainty in the neighborhood as the college undertook expansion. Even the museums of the cultural district were overwhelmed by their new—and growing—neighbor. "They were overshadowed," Coffelt explains. It was a matter of height. At eight stories and set on a hill, Med Ed I towered over the museums. It had been designed, however, to complement the existing architecture of the museums, and today they are good neighbors.

There was some disagreement on the location of the second building on TCOM's campus. Some wanted it in Denton; Willard reminded them that the state charter specified a medical school in Tarrant County. Then there were proposals to locate it in far north Tarrant County, nearly halfway to Denton. The issue was settled in 1979 when Representative Gib Lewis introduced a bill authorizing the school to acquire land in its own neighborhood.

LaRue was made responsible for acquisition of the necessary land, an unpleasant job which meant evicting neighbors from the small homes that surrounded the college. The legislature had allocated three-and-a-half million dollars to buy land and had changed the statute to allow the state to buy land for TCOM. (Under the original agreement, TCOM was to be located at a site in Tarrant Country provided at no cost to the state). But the Board of Regents decreed that the college could not pay above appraised value for any of the land. It made LaRue's job difficult, but not impossible.

"Some of our neighbors—most of them intelligent people— knew how to build a backfire. They went to the local radio stations, local TV stations, local newspapers, and told them that LaRue was trying to steal from them." TV crews would come out and set up cameras, but the college kept the message going that they wanted to be fair about appraisals.

Once, LaRue recalls, a man and his son came to his office with the expressed intent of beating him up. "I demonstrated my skill then at talking, and I talked them out of doing that." About a year later, the college bought their property, and the family settled in a new home in Fort Worth. When the parents celebrated their fiftieth wedding anniversay, LaRue was an honored guest at the party.

In all, the college dealt with twenty-two property owners and purchased each piece at appraised value, without invoking the right of eminent domain and condemnation of property.

The college leaders persuaded the city to close a block-long side

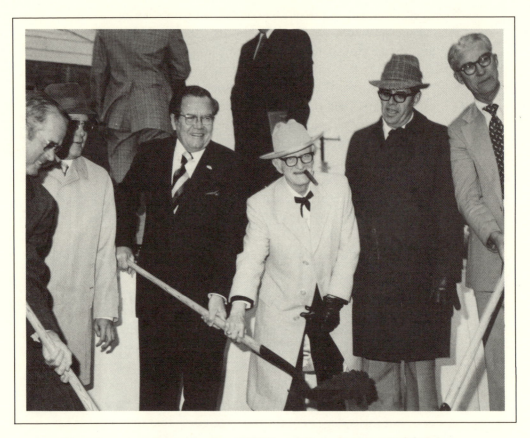

November, 1976: dignitaries from NTSU and Texas Governor Dolph Briscoe celebrate ground breaking for Med Ed I.

street that the present building sits right on. Construction began in 1981, and again, under the supervision of Mike Miller, the building was completed ahead of schedule. The five-story "Med Ed II," at a cost of sixteen million dollars, was more expensive because more plumbing and intricate construction were required for the research facilities it houses; in addition, construction costs had risen since the building of Med Ed I. Med Ed II, occupied in the fall of 1982, contains basic science departments, kiva and panoramic classrooms, and research laboratories. With its completion, the college was able to bring together all basic science teaching and research in one area. It was a major step forward for TCOM.

In the 1983 legislative session, money was appropriated for the third major building, "Med Ed III," planned as a medical library. A committee from TCOM visited other libraries, particularly health sciences libraries, throughout the state, taking with them representatives from Fisher and Spillman, the same architectural firm that had designed Med Ed I and II. Meanwhile, back home, college officials were fighting off an attempt to locate an M.D. program in Tarrant County and have the two programs share the facilities of Med Ed II.

"In my opinion," says Willard, "that would have simply diluted the educational program and not benefited anyone in Texas." Eventually, though, construction funds were caught by depressed economic conditions in Texas and legislative concern over the expenditure of funds. Willard persisted, and groundbreaking for the third building was held in September 1984.

Although the same architects had been employed for Med Ed III, a new contractor was used—Sogetex, an international company with main offices in France but branch headquarters in Dallas. They were low bidders on the job and were awarded the contract. But it soon became known that once they finished Med Ed III they intended to close their U.S. office due to declining construction activity in this country.

Coffelt asked the company not to make that fact known, fearing difficulties with deliveries. Instead, the company went public with their anticipated removal from the U.S., and difficulties followed almost immediately—the project went over budget and behind schedule. There was a constant quality battle between the college and the contractors. It was a difficult period, one not to be repeated, but the building was finally completed to the satisfaction of college officials and occupied in December 1986.

Med Ed III, costing fourteen million dollars, is perhaps the most dramatic of the three major campus buildings. Built on a natural slope, it features large expanses of bronze glass, with a spectacular view of Fort Worth's skyline, open balconies, and a two-story atrium. The building houses the Health Sciences Library, with room for the expansion inevitable in a library, a state-of-the-art biomedical communications department, a computing services department, and a computer classroom.

In its history, the TCOM library has endured several moves—a major undertaking for any library. From the fifth floor of FWOH to the bowling alley/administration building to the River Plaza building, then to the seventh floor of Med Ed I. By that time, the collection had reached 35,000 volumes and there was a staff of twenty-seven, including Bobby R. Carter, the new library director. When the library moved into its permanent quarters in Med Ed III, the move involved about 90,000 volumes, a journal collection approaching 2,300 titles, and 3,500 audiovisual titles—all valued at near four and a half million dollars—and a staff of over forty.

The library, one of the most advanced medical libraries in the Southwest, is a center for medical information for Fort Worth and Tarrant County. Virtually all of the world's current medical information is available to students, physicians and the community through TCOM's sophisticated computer-search systems and communications network. Information from any of 200 data bases nationwide can be accessed within a matter of seconds, then viewed, mailed or transmitted by telefacsimile. The Library's rare book and special collections are in a specially designed space with lighted display cases, fire security, and climate controls to provide proper maintenance and storage of a collection of volumes and memorabilia dealing mostly with osteopathic medical history and nineteenth-century American medicine.

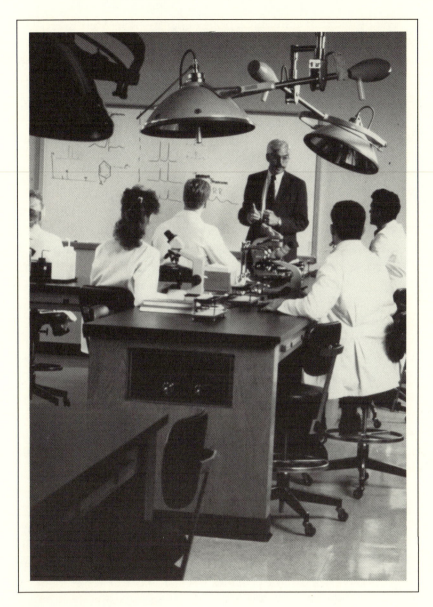

Lab scene, 1990.

The biomedical communications department in Med Ed III also represents the finest in equipment and services. It was not always so. Coffelt, who was director of educational television at Tarrant County Junior College, remembers when he was hired to start a biomedical communications department at TCOM. Marion Coy, then-president of TCOM, visited Coffelt on the TCJC campus; Coffelt, thinking Coy wanted to see their facilities which had by then gained national reputation, gave him a tour of their learning resources center. But Coy was more direct: "Would you like to go to work for me?" he asked. Coffelt agreed to visit.

"I walked into a bowling alley," he recalls. He was shown the space alloted for an instructional media department—three rooms in the back of Central Clinic. "I was coming from one of the most modern, up-to-date media delivery systems in the country at that time," says Coffelt, "but I liked the challenge of starting from scratch." Coffelt, whose degree was in biology, also liked the idea of medicine. He showed up for work on January 2, 1974.

Today the biomedical communications department is, according to Coffelt, "one of the best in the Southwest in an institution of this size." TCOM is recognized nationally for leadership in medical informatics—the application of computer technology to medical education, research and practice. In addition, the department provides services in graphic arts, photography, television production, audio tapes, visual projects such as transparencies and slides, medical illustration, biomedical instrumentation repair and bioelectronics.

For eleven years, from 1975 until 1986, the college was almost continually under construction, with at best two year gaps between building programs. Today the three pre-cast concrete buildings dominate the campus, but there are other buldings—an Activity Center, built in a former Mormon tabernacle, sits on the northern edge of the campus and provides over 12,000 feet for student activities and the public health and preventive medicine department. Campus police are housed in a small building on Camp Bowie, and the department of medical humanities occupies a charming rock house, built in 1929, at the far edge of the campus. The medicine

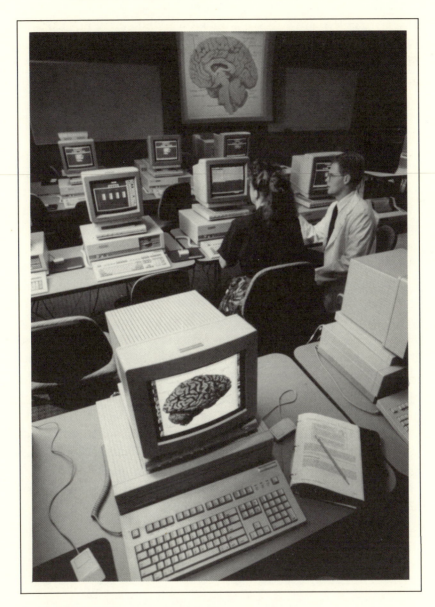

Inside Med Ed III—computer technology at work.

and surgery departments have their own clinic buildings fronting on Montgomery, and there is a physical plant headquarters.

The campus of slightly over fifteen acres is not large, but it's sufficient to educate 400 physicians. The buildings are surrounded by parking lots, but here and there they boast an inviting bench, a scenic bit of landscaping. Basically, it is a sleek, modern campus, and it speaks well for the institution which it houses.

Thinking back on the college's building phase, Willard says "People and programs are more important than buildings, but perhaps I underestimate the importance of buildings. . . . It shows up in our student recruiting efforts and, even more so, in our faculty recruiting efforts. . . . Once that building [Med Ed I] started coming out of the ground, recruiting became infinitely easier, and we have been able to go out and get people and develop programs with these buildings."

In 1990, a campus master plan indicates ways in which the campus can be expanded; space is already at a critical premium, and plans are on the drawing board to expand clinical operations into property on Camp Bowie Boulevard. The college's clinics are growing rapidly and the research programs expanding; both require space.

TCOM, with a modern, efficient and breathtaking campus, looks to a future of physical growth, even with the inevitable restrictions of an inner city campus. In part, the college has growing pains because it is in a central, populated area. But it needs to be in just such an area to have a constituency to serve and a hospital affiliation.

৯৯৯ *Goals and Signposts*

W HEN AN INSTITUTION IS YOUNG, ITS SIGNPOSTS TEND TO BE clearcut and obvious—a first class, a new building, something tangible. As it grows and its programs become more complex, signposts may be more difficult to mark. They may represent giant steps, but they are often steps recognized only by those within the institutional community.

For TCOM, three significant goal statements have been such signposts. The first, issued in March 1980, dealt with the educational curriculum.

In 1977 the Curriculum Committee recommended that the college needed a working document which expressed specific objectives for the institution's educational program. The committee at that time was chaired by Dr. Charles Ogilvie. After consultation with the administration, Ogilvie recommended the establishment of a blue-ribbon task force to develop a working document containing the college's goals. Ogilvie appointed a committee, including Dr. I. M. Korr, who was asked by TCOM President Ralph Willard to chair the task force.

Korr, a physiologist, was known as a major contributor to modern scientific understanding of the osteopathic profession. A faculty member of the Kirksville college for many years, he was the first scientific researcher to study osteopathic principles and to relate the results of his research to the clinical practice of osteopathic medicine. By the mid-1970s, he was renowned throughout the profession not only for his scientific knowledge and accomplishments but for his insight into the special problems of osteopathic education. He had left Kirksville to join the faculty of the Michigan College of Osteopathic Medicine and then, with the encouragement of Ogilvie, joined the TCOM faculty because of the great potential he saw in the Texas institution.

Korr's initial response to Willard's invitation was that he had participated in the writing of too many pompous manifestos, "filled with pious platitudes that nobody could disagree with [but] had no impact whatsoever. . . . I didn't want to resume that activity anymore." Assured that this was to be a working document with enormous impact on the college, he accepted the challenge to develop goals for osteopathic medical education that were appropriate to the times and to our culture, especially to the State of Texas.

The Task Force on Educational Goals, with Korr as chairman, was formed in October 1978. Other members were Drs. Richard Baldwin, Russell Gamber, Elizabeth Harris, C. Raymond Olson, and Jay Shores, along with student doctor Eric Simmons (Class of 1980). Ogilvie, as the one who had instigated the project and shares major credit for its successful completion, was an ex-officio member of the committee, attending all meetings in his position as chair of the curriculum committee.

Korr asked the task force to begin with a basic question: Why are there two complete schools of medicine, two distinct professions? He suggested that the only reason for the existence of any profession is that it meets needs not met by any other occupation. Then, he suggested, the question which follows is, "Are there any unmet needs in American health care?" There was, he recalls, stunned silence. "Scientists," he explains, "are reluctant to consider this possibility."

The task force met for eight months, meeting several hours weekly, attempting to define the educational goals of the college in relation to society's health-care needs. In essence, the committee studied health care in America. Eventually it became clear that there were gaps in the system, inequities and unsolved problems to be addressed. As one member of the team said, "It was like finding that your mother isn't quite a lady to discover that American medicine isn't everything it's been touted to be."

"What we were seeing," Korr says, "was that the health-care system was totally absorbed in dealing with established disease, mostly the chronic degenerative diseases which were not like infectious diseases—something you catch one day and become sick the next. These are the products, the culmination of whole lifetimes; therefore, the only hope was to move upstream and catch the early departures from health, even better than that to promote and enhance health. The premise is that the healthier you are, the less likely you are to become sick."

The task force divided into groups, each assigned specific jobs. One of them, according to Korr, was to define the scope of the osteopathic movement in medicine. Another was to describe the behaviors of a physician who would achieve these health-related goals—things like being a self-starter, an effective problem-solver, someone who would intiate programs and activities. In the end, the task force presented the philosophy that preventive medicine must become the core of medical education, replacing the old-style episodic medicine and its concentration on disease.

The approach was, of course, the philosophy of Andrew Taylor Still, founder of osteopathic medicine. "Preventive medicine themes permeate [Still's] writings and are an integral part of his teaching," explains Ralph Willard. "Osteopathic diagnosis and treatment by musculoskeletal means reduce the dependence on drugs and surgery and, of course, if started early enough, can prevent late-stage surgery. . . . The goals statement is an osteopathic document."

The statement recommended transfer of emphasis from therapy to prevention, from late-stage disease to early departure from health. It stressed the need for the patient to take responsibility for his own health care, the need for health education for patients, the need for physicians to serve as role models of wellness lifestyle and prevention, and the need for more emphasis on preventive nutrition in medical schools.

In a tentative look at implementation, the task force recommended changes in curricular content (the curriculum had been

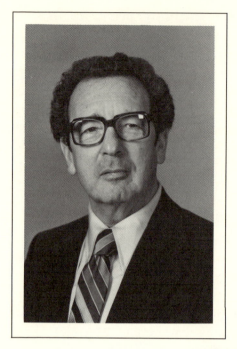

I. M. Korr.

Charles Ogilvie.

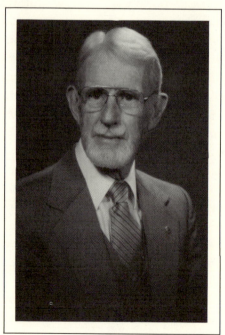

virtually unchanged since the first year), clinical experiences for students, faculty approaches to teaching, and the criteria for selection of students.

The NTSU board of regents and Chancellor Frank E. Vandiver, as well as the TCOM president, went on record supporting the goals statement. Willard notes that many people hailed the statement as a new document, "a forerunner of the twenty-first century medical school." He sees it equally as a return to the principles that caused the creation of the first college of osteopathic medicine. Following the 1980 publication of the goals statement, documents published by the U.S. Department of Health and Human Services put new emphasis on preventive medicine and a report called GPEP—General Professional Education of the Physician for the Twenty-first Century—issued by the American Association of Medical Schools in 1984 reinforced the concepts of the TCOM goals statement. TCOM's educational program was on the leading edge of changing thought in modern medicine.

The educational goals statement encouraged TCOM to take a leadership role in health and prevention matters. The school was, for instance, one of the first institutions to declare itself a totally smoke-free environment. No smoking is permitted anywhere on the campus. When the policy was instituted in October 1987, the college received a commendation from the U.S. Surgeon General for its smoke-free policy.

The goals statement called particular attention to nutrition, a field not usually given prominence in medical education. Through an endowment from UNT Regent E. Bruce Street, Sr., and his wife, the college recognizes outstanding contributions in this field with the Roger J. Williams Award in Preventive Nutrition. By 1989 the award had been presented five times, most recently to Bruce N. Ames, a professor of biochemistry at the University of California at Berkeley, who developed an important laboratory test which searches for possible cancer-causing agents in food and drugs. The Williams award includes an honorarium, and the recpient presents a public lecture at TCOM.

The Institute for Human Fitness represents another implemen-

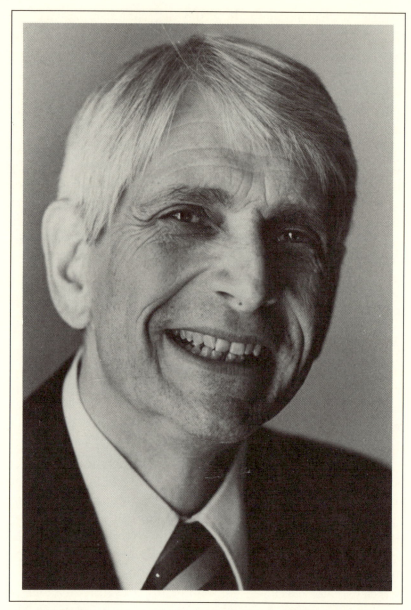

Frank E. Vandiver, Ph.D., who served TCOM as president for fifteen months between 1979 and 1981. Vandiver, whose academic specialty is military history, participated in the development of TCOM's statement of clinical goals.

tation of the principles of the goals statement. The idea for the institute came from casual conversation between Ogilvie and Dr. Robert Kaman of the biochemistry department. They gathered several other interested faculty members—all marathon runners—and began meeting on Sunday afternoons in the home of general surgeon Joel Alter. What grew out of these conversations was an exercise-centered program for persons whose health was on the wellness end of the health/disease continuum.

The Institute of Human Fitness was created in 1978 and housed in the River Plaza facility of the campus, conveniently located near the Trinity River jogging and bike trail, and by 1979 it had expanded to become a health and fitness center for the community. The "healthy patient" was given a thorough health and fitness assessment followed by an individualized prescription for exercise, nutrition or behavioral change. Individuals undergoing rehabilitation from athletic, work or illness-related injury were introduced into the program under the supervision of a physical therapist or an athletic trainer.

Operating on a membership basis, the institute offered wellness assessments, individualized exercise programs, and support for such other college programs as cardiac rehabilitation. In addition, it provided such services as a physical fitness program for the Fort Worth Fire Department and a program for the Star House Alcohol Recovery Center. The institute became best known, however, for originating the Cowtown Marathon, Fort Worth's 26.2-mile race co-sponsored since 1978 by TCOM, the *Fort Worth Star-Telegram*, and, in more recent years, Miller Brewing Company and the Osteopathic Medical Center of Texas. Today the race enjoys a reputation as one of the best-managed road races of its kind in Texas with over 8,000 runners participating in either the marathon or the associated 10-K race.

Although several health and fitness centers for the "healthy patient" are available in Fort Worth now, there were few in the late seventies when the institute began operation. In 1987, the state restricted funds available to state agencies for the rental of property and the institute was formally dissolved, though its functions are ongoing within the college in the Activity Center and the department of public health and preventive medicine.

The impact of the goals statement was also apparent in the orientation of entering students. In the mid-seventies, several faculty members were keenly aware of the personal strain placed on students. A "survival course" emerged. The course, utilizing some of the theories behind Outward Bound courses, was designed to give incoming students a set of skills to allow them to carry the stress of medical school without resorting to destructive behavior. A highlight of that early orientation course was the "healthy" breakfasts planned and served by Ogilvie's wife Reva. The survival course has today evolved into a series of interdisciplinary workshops, now offered by the department of medical humanities, that look at stress management for both students and physicians.

A second signpost statement was adopted in November 1984, dealing with the research goals of the college. Osteopathic medicine and scientific research were for many years uneasy companions, and the profession tended to dedicate itself more to clinical service than to research. The osteopathic philosophy and its implementation in practice did not lend themselves easily to the measurement of traditional scientific methods. And D.O.s have traditionally not been prolific writers. Research scientists were generally attracted to established allopathic medical institutions with proven records of extramural funding.

For all these reasons, establishing a research program in a new medical school is a major challenge; establishing one in an osteopathic medical school is an adventure fraught with impossibilities. Yet from the beginning, TCOM's founders and administrators recognized that just as a university strives for a well-rounded program, a medical school must contribute in all the academic arenas of health care, including biomedical research. When the completion of the three major buildings provided state-of-the-art research facilities, expanded library services, and biomedical communications services—all of which made the college more attractive to highly qualified research scientists—it was time to examine the direction of the research program.

The research goals statement, in harmony with the educational goals statement, puts emphasis on health, viewing it as not merely the absence of disease but a phenomenon in itself, the appropriate subject of research. The statement recommends that physiological mechanisms inherent in health, the musculoskeletal system and its interplay with other systems, and osteopathic methods of diagnosis and therapy were appropriate primary areas of research for the college.

Specifically, the statement calls for an increase in research publications and scientific presentations by the faculty, an increase in extramural funding for research, an increase in interaction between the basic and clinical sciences, and expansion of graduate and other programs in conjunction with several departments at North Texas State University. The administration was challenged to provide not only the physical facilities necessary to foster scientific endeavor but also to "encourage and reward meaningful research" by requiring it for tenure and promotion, implementing a reward system, supporting efforts to gain extramural funding, and supporting efforts to make the public aware of important health-related research being conducted at TCOM.

Ultimately, though, as in the educational goals statement, the challenge was to the faculty to develop individual projects that paralleled the goals of the college and to assume final responsibility for the success of the research program at TCOM.

The significance of the research goals statement is that it supports the clinical goals statement, providing the data to support what osteopathic physicians have always believed intuitively about wellness and the quality of life.

The final goals statement, adopted in June 1987, was one of responsibility to the community and to the osteopathic profession. Community service has always been a key part of osteopathic medicine; in Fort Worth, the profession had established a record of community service long before the establishment of TCOM. From the first, expansion of this community-service role was essential to the overall program at TCOM.

The goals statement on community service recognizes the importance of service to the general welfare of the community as well as its potential for the exchange of knowledge. In addition to community service, it stresses service to professional organizations and continuing medical education. Most importantly, it recognizes community service as an essential part of the educational program of a physician.

"Community service," says Dr. Virginia Ellis, former director of the program, "has three purposes: One is to [get students] to look at their own attitudes, because they are [in] a helping profession and they need to know . . . how they are going to feel as doctors dealing with alcohol, drugs, the handicapped, the retarded, and geriatrics. . . . The second goal is to have a student doctor become familiar with the various agencies and services available to him as a physician and to his patients. . . . He is part of a team and there are lots of people out there who are well trained to help him in the care of his patients. The third goal is for the student doctor to give of himself by providing free services that will make him a part of a community."

These three goals statements, issued over a span of seven years, define the areas of emphasis at TCOM: education, research, community service. It's a three-pronged program with one major mission: the education of osteopathic physicians to provide health care for the people of Texas and the United States.

There have been other signposts along the way as the college grew and matured. One was the creation in May 1981 of the position of president of the college, with the stipulation that the president would always be an osteopathic physician and would be responsible to the Board of Regents of the University of North Texas through the chancellor who served both institutions. Until that time, the chief executive officer at TCOM had been a dean. Chancellor Al Hurley calls this administrative reorganization a major signpost in the evolution of TCOM's organizational structure.

Ralph Willard was the first president to serve directly under a chancellor from NTSU. When he left office in 1985, he was succeeded as interim president by Dr. David Richards, who had previously been dean for academic affairs. An osteopathic general practitioner,

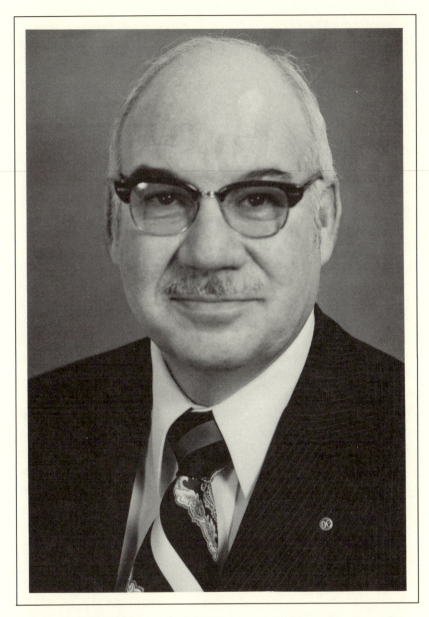

Ralph L. Willard, D.O., dean from 1975 to 1980 and president from 1981 to 1985. During his tenure, the college adopted its statement of research goals, and the physical plant grew dramatically with the opening of Med Ed I and II and the beginning of construction for Med Ed III.

Richards had previously been associate dean for academic and clinical affairs and founding chairman of the department of family medicine at Ohio University College of Osteopathic Medicine. Richards brought with him strong consultant experience working with the U.S. Department of Health, Education and Welfare, the National Fund for Medical Education, and other colleges of osteopathic medicine. A past president of the Ohio Society of General Practitioners, Richards began his professional career in general practice in Ohio. Clearly, he was and is an administrator who emphasizes the college's mandate to produce general practitioners.

Another signpost, according to both Hurley and Richards, was the statement known as "Thirty-Nine Points," issued in 1984. It is, says Richards, a restatement of the original goals statement on the curriculum. "We were in deep straits in 1984," he explains. "We took students who were wonderful people but didn't have the MCAT (Medical College Aptitude Test) score or the GPA (grade point average) to handle the medical licensure examination. What had been a failure rate of eleven or twelve percent became twenty-one percent, and the board of regents and the legislature wanted to know why."

The academic standards of the college, particularly in the admissions policies, were raised. "It was a major point of controversy among the osteopathic profession," admits Richards, "but it was upheld by the board of regents. We cannot afford to be sentimental and admit someone's son or nephew or neighbor just because they've loved osteopathic medicine all their lives. They have to have the appropriate background and test scores."

This policy meant strengthening the efforts toward minority recruitment at a time when the national pool of medical school applicants was shrinking, particularly among the minorities. Among other programs, TCOM put into action a strong minority assistance program to help qualified students meet the academic standards for admission.

The Thirty-Nine Points statement was effective. All 1988 graduates who took the Federal Licensure Examination (FLEX) passed, their scores the culmination of a steady improvement in FLEX scores that began in 1984, the first year of implementation of the Thirty-Nine Points.

In 1987, a select committee of the Texas committee on higher education undertook a major investigation of state supported health schools. Along with medical, dental and nursing schools, they looked at TCOM: another signpost. "We went up a level in the tiering of schools," says Richards. "There was a better understanding with other schools, a better understanding in the legislature of our programs, a better understanding that we have a unique perspective in relation to other schools. That inspection was a major stepping stone, the single most important factor in our increased recognition within the state."

One result of this increased recognition was a fourteen percent budget increase in the 1989–90 fiscal year, higher than any other medical school. Another was that TCOM was asked to be part of the paternity testing network in the state. Richards explains that there is far-reaching research potential in DNA testing which is done to determine paternity; it may well lead to diagnostic and treatment methods for some cancers and it has proven important in criminal investigations.

Two major signposts involved strengthening the facilities for clinical training. In 1988, TCOM entered into an arrangement with Carswell Air Force Base in Fort Worth to provide clinical outpatient care for retired personnel. In essence, the school committed to a partnership which traded service for educational opportunity. In 1989, a similar arrangement was reached with the Veterans Administrations Central Administration Office of Academic Affairs to provide care at the Bonham, Texas, center. "The osteopathic profession does not have a long history of these affiliations," said Richards. "They've come about because we're now recognized as a national figure in medical circles. We're a player in the system."

In 1989, the college issued an economic impact statement, subtitled "A Report to Our Community," showing that the college provides employment directly or indirectly for over 2,000 people; local banks enjoy more than eleven million dollars in additional deposits;

local business volume is increased by more than fifty million dollars; total personal income in the area is increased by more than thirty million dollars. The people who work at TCOM make significant contributions to the health and prosperity of Fort Worth, Tarrant County, and the State of Texas.

Still another signpost: In 1989, with a $1.1 million grant from the Kellogg Foundation, TCOM received its first support from a major private foundation outside of Texas and Oklahoma. "It took some planning," says Richards. "A wellness and prevention proposal did not work, but when we proposed a community-oriented primary-care project, they were interested and made site visits." The grant is to be given on a matching basis, with the college challenged to raise funds within the state. The project will begin on Fort Worth's North Side. "It will be an inner city research program," says Richards. "We can influence health care delivery significantly. Take hypertension, diabetes, AIDS, whatever, and involve the community through awareness. . . . The grant is a major step for the college."

In recent years, the signposts seem to have come one upon the heels of another as the college gains state and national recognition and its programs expand in importance and complexity. Twenty years ago few would have dared envision the enviable record of accomplishment that is today the history of TCOM.

ஐஐ *The Clinical Program*

Dᴀᴠɪᴅ Rᴀʏ sᴘᴏᴋᴇ ғᴏʀ ᴀʟʟ ᴍᴇᴅɪᴄᴀʟ sᴛᴜᴅᴇɴᴛs ᴡʜᴇɴ ʜᴇ sᴀɪᴅ, "Every medical student wants to get to a patient. From the day he arrives, he wants to get to a living, breathing thing. . . . Even when he gets to see his first patient, that isn't enough. He wants to do more and more. . . ." Clinical training is indeed the pinnacle of a medical student's experience. At ᴛᴄᴏᴍ, the clinical program has grown and developed, influenced by the goals statement, and given depth by the osteopathic concern for the patient as a potentially healthy human being.

During the college's first year of operation, Dr. Joel Alter, a general surgeon, reluctantly took over the job of clinical coordinator, comparable today to the position of clinical dean, on the condition that it was a temporary position. He would receive no money, and his recommendations would be subject to approval by the board since he was acutely aware of his lack of background for the position. "There was no clinical program," he explains. "The students were busy with the basic sciences, but we needed a curriculum for accreditation purposes." Alter got catalogs from osteopathic and allopathic medical schools and, with the help of a committee, created a paper curriculum.

Dr. Ray Olson, former chair of the department of internal medicine, recalls that "Dr. Tom Whittle lectured that first year on the psychology of normal behavior." Whittle was a general practitioner with a strong interest in pscyhology. "He lectured in the garage apartment, and that was the only clinical instruction the students got their first year."

The second year, Dr. John Kemplin agreed to teach a course in his specialty, radiology, to give the students some clinical exposure, and Olson instituted weekly grand rounds in internal medicine, ninety-minute sessions which focused on a new clinical problem each week. Since the sessions used live patients, problem selection pretty much depended on the availability of patients, according to Olson. "It wasn't an attempt to cover everything, but we worked to introduce a different kind of pathology each week." Students were still heavily involved with basic science education in their sophmore year, Olson remembers.

As the first class approached the end of their second year, however, it was apparent that the clinical program needed structure. The development of the internal medicine curriculum is fairly typical of the development of clinical programs at the college. George Luibel asked Olson to put together a curriculum for internal medicine, and Olson's first move was to arrange a meeting of area internists in Arlington.

"We looked at the standard texts and were overwhelmed," says Olson, "so I called George Luibel to ask what the thrust of the medical school experience should be."

The answer he received was "Teach what should be taught in medical school." They divided the textbook into sections, and various internists, all volunteer, each took a section as their responsibility. By 1972, there was a clinical curriculum with an established lecture program. "Sometimes we filled in with local M.D.s," says Olson. "They were the first ones to be paid."

The early clinical program at TCOM was one of educating physicians as well as students. "We were teaching physicians to teach," explains Alter. "We had to establish the training of doctors to become teachers, as well as the training of students to become doctors." Olson, for example, recalls teaching a course in pulmonary medicine; he had gone off campus about a month earlier to take a course in pulmonary medicine himself to prepare for his teaching experience. "But," repeats Alter, "it was more than learning to teach the basics of medicine. We had to learn to be teachers."

In late fall, Ray Olson accepted a fifty percent annual salary to be dean of clinical sciences. After three months, he saw that the arrangement wasn't working. "The board was honest in what they wanted to do and also honest in squarely facing their fiscal limitations," says Olson, "but I had a family to support and educate, and I couldn't do it on a half-time private practice."

In 1972, the students also began daylong clinical clerkship rotations at various area osteopathic hospitals. The clerkships began as experiences in clinical observation and only gradually evolved into positions where students could participate in the care of a patient. But it was soon obvious that someone needed to direct the clinical rotation program. An inspection program was needed to ensure the quality of the educational experience the students got in each hospital. "Sometimes they were seen as free labor," Olson explains, "and we had to avoid that." Olson, as volunteer chairman of the department, could not undertake the inspection program; he had a private practice to maintain and a family to support.

Olson was followed by Dr. Joe DePetris, a Dallas internist who had been one of the original group planning the medicine curriculum. DePetris extended the clinical rotations to include lectures and sent students to the hospitals for a week at a time.

When Dr. Edward T. (Ned) Newell joined the faculty in January 1973, he assumed the duties of the clinical dean, although he was hired as an academic dean and, in February 1973, given the official title of vice-president for academic affairs by the board of directors. As such, he took over many of Hardt's duties, who, preparing to retire, stayed on in a different capacity. Newell, former director of medical education at Metropolitan Hospital in Philadelphia and a physician with a long record of medical teaching, served as vice-president for two years and then as associate dean for the clinical sciences. He left the college about a year after Ralph Willard's arrival.

In 1975, Willard, newly hired as dean, in turn hired Olson as full-time chairman of the department of internal medicine. The department had no other full-time faculty and continued to use local osteopathic physicians, augmented by M.D.s, for lectures in the subspecialties. Faculty from the University of Texas Southwestern Medical School in Dallas frequently served as visiting lecturers until 1979 or 1980 when the state ruled that they could not be paid for lecturing, since they were already on the state payroll as faculty at a medical college.

The first two additional full-time faculty members in the department of medicine were hired in 1976, though neither stayed long at the college. "Private practice was always more lucrative, expecially for those who don't get the satisfaction out of teaching that some of us do," Olson explains. "Some are teachers, some are not."

A few full-time faculty joined other departments—Earle F. Starkey in pathology, for instance—but the first big wave did not come until 1975 and 1976. Several came from Michigan State University College of Osteopathic Medicine, where they had worked directly with Willard, and most of these were members of the department of general practice. Although TCOM had graduated one class and enrolled five, it had few full-time faculty up until that time, and students were going all over to study. Interestingly enough, although almost all the osteopathic teaching hospitals in Texas were then and are now located in the Dallas-Fort Worth area—Corpus Christi and Groves are exceptions—there were not enough standard rotations available locally.

Clerkships, according to Dr. Richard Baldwin, former associate dean for clinical studies, prepare the student for internship. The American Osteopathic Association requires a rotating internship following graduation; whereas students in M.D. schools often declare their area of specialty by the fourth year, osteopathic students are required to be "generalists" through their internship. The requirement is part of the profession's emphasis on general practice and family medicine, but it imposes difficulties on a medical school—difficulties that involve affiliating with sufficient training institutions.

"With one hundred students needing to spend a month in medicine, a month in surgery, some time in pediatrics and obstetrics, and with two or three hospitals, it's impossible," says Baldwin. "The ratio of cases and teaching physicians simply isn't enough." As a result, students went all over the country, particularly to such states as Ohio, Michigan and Missouri which have a much longer history of osteopathic teaching hospitals than Texas.

But in Texas there was strong effort to build up the teaching affiliations with the metroplex hospitals, and by about 1982 the college was able to place all its students in approved clerkships in local hospitals. Participating osteopathic hospitals were East Town Osteopathic Hospital, Dallas Family Hospital and Dallas Memorial, Northeast Community in Hurst, and Dallas/Fort Worth Medical Center, Grand Prairie. "When they're close by, we can monitor the quality of the educational experience," says Baldwin, "and we can support the hospital better with a close relationship. The college provides a secretary for the clerkship program, and we contribute to the library fund, things like that."

In addition to area osteopathic institutions, the college has clerkship programs at William Beaumont Army Medical Center in El Paso, Corpus Christi Osteopathic Hospital, the hospital at Carswell Air Force Base in Fort Worth, and the University of Texas Health Center at Tyler. In addition, students can and do arrange elective rotations at AMA accredited hospitals.

Physicians who oversee rotations in these various institutions are unpaid but have clinical faculty status at the college. Generally, the relationshp is a mutually beneficial one, with students given educational exposure to hospital practice and physicians benefitting from the teaching experience while their hospitals benefit from the work done by clinical clerks. Supervising physicians often visit campus, and they are appreciative of the support provided by TCOM facilities like the library.

The Osteopathic Medical Center of Texas is the primary teaching hospital and the majority of students do most of their rotations at that 265-bed institution. "For its size," says Baldwin, "Fort Worth O. offers an incredibly rich depth and array of specialists—and this

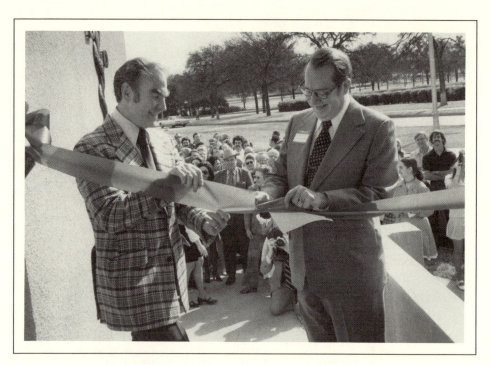

U. S. Representative Jim Wright, left, holds a ribbon for Dr. George Luibel to cut with a scalpel during opening ceremonies of the college's second outpatient clinic at 3440 Camp Bowie, Fort Worth. Below, the Justin Clinic.

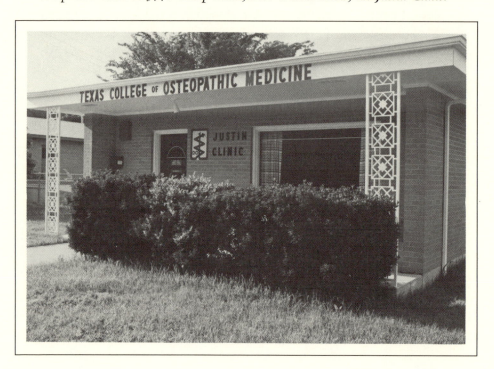

is due in part to its affiliation with a medical school." Baldwin explains that because of its specialty staff, the hospital takes care of more complex cases—"the level of illness is higher"—thereby justifying an intensity of diagnostic and therapeutic care that students do not necessarily get in affiliated clerkship programs.

Increasingly each year, a good percentage of the medical center's staff physicians are TCOM graduates. They may have stayed right after graduation or they may have gone elsewhere for advanced training and returned, but they come back because they like Fort Worth and because they were treated well as students at the center. "It's important that we see that their training experience at our hospital is positive," says Jay Sandelin, Osteopathic Medical Center of Texas chairman of the board and CEO. "Then they'll come back to augment our staff."

The relationship between the college and OMCT has been a necessarily close one for years, but also one which both institutions work hard to maintain. Together the two form an osteopathic community, a highly visible presence not only in the Cultural District but in the city at large. Inevitably they are linked as one institution in the public mind, though they are separate and totally independent. Still, what affects one affects the other, for they represent osteopathic medicine in Fort Worth.

And there are tangible links. TCOM President David Richards serves as an ad hoc member of the OMCT board of trustees; Sandelin, a layman, got his first introduction to osteopathic medicine when he was asked to join the board of the then-private TCOM in the early seventies. Today he is chairman of the TCOM Advisory Council and a member of several national osteopathic committees.

Speaking of the early days of the clerkship program at FWOH, Olson says "There was ardent bedside teaching, but there were holes in the program." One of the holes was a lack of coordination between the medical and surgical departments. The first chair of the department of surgery was Dr. Nat Stewart of Mid-Cities Memorial Osteopathic Hospital; his vice-chairman was Joel Alter, who had been clinical coordinator. Alter describes that early teaching program as one of a highly traditional format, with lectures from various surgeons and a surgical text for students.

But students were viewing one disease entity from at least two viewponts—that of the surgeon and that of the internist. Gradually the two departments moved into a sort of co-teaching. When the thyroid was studied, a surgeon sat in on the medicine lectures. There was what Olson terms "dialog teaching." It was, he says, incredibly innovative and courageous.

"We moved toward matrix management," he explains, "which says that the most important thing is the program, not the department. You use people from whatever discipline is necessary to build the program. But matrix management represents a departure from traditional academia, which is built on departments not programs. Funding is generally done on the basis of departments. It's difficult to change the entire academic structure."

As the medical and surgical departments began to merge their teaching programs, the problem-oriented approach of a New England physician named Lawrence Weed was incorporated. Actually, Weed's approach had been introduced by Olson as early as 1972, but it was later given greater emphasis by the curriculum committee which was headed by Ogilvie, a strong believer in Weed's method. Weed's contribution of problem-oriented record-keeping, sometimes called one of the most revolutionary concepts in modern medical education, provides for longitudinal patient records organized according to a problem list. Each individual's problem list is different, according to the state of their health and the factors that are part of their overall health condition. The physician views the patient's presenting complaint in the context of the individual's entire health picture. In American medicine generally, such longitudinal records are not kept; each visit to the doctor is a brand new experience. The longitudinal record, by tracking health factors in each individual, facilitates the practice of preventive medicine. "It guides your thinking," says Olson, "and reinforces the osteopathic idea of looking at the whole patient. It also focuses attention on the patient's problem, rather than the doctor's particular interest."

A second major influence was the medical education program at

McMaster University in Ontario, a program replacing rote memorization with creative thinking, utilizing what was called problem-solving learning.

"We were looking for innovative teaching for excellence," says Olson. "What we arrived at was that we would not teach the students medicine, but we would teach them to teach themselves medicine. I was aided by a creative student who said, 'I am my own medical school. I am primarily responsible for my own teaching and learning.'"

In problem-solving learning, an organ is studied from every vantage point, with basic scientists and clinicians working together cooperatively. Medicine is studied by systems instead of disciplines such as medicine, surgery, and so on. "We moved dramatically away from tradition," says Olson, noting that in 1979 there were no traditional lectures; in 1980, a handful; in 1981, a few more. By 1983, the program was back to the more traditional one dominated by lectures, but the problem-solving methods left an indelible impact.

Just as some are teachers and some aren't, not all faculty are adept at problem-solving teaching, nor do all students find it the optimum way to learn. "It's difficult to train faculty to become tutors. In problem-solving learning, they do not dispense knowledge. But they *must* watch the students like a hawk, they must listen creatively and comment. There is no more money, no reward beyond the appreciation of the students."

Problem-solving learning became an integral part of the clinical program at TCOM, though the clinical curriculum is still organized along the traditional lines of medical disciplines. Olson sees the college as undeniably affected by the goals statement as well as problem-solving approaches, both of which have contributed to create a distinctive curriculum. "We made mistakes in the past which we must pay for," he concludes, "but the future is good. We must not let go of our osteopathic nature. We must appreciate the difference."

The department of medical humanities represents another innovative approach to clinical education at TCOM. Formed in the late 1970s, it was one of only a dozen or so such departments in medical

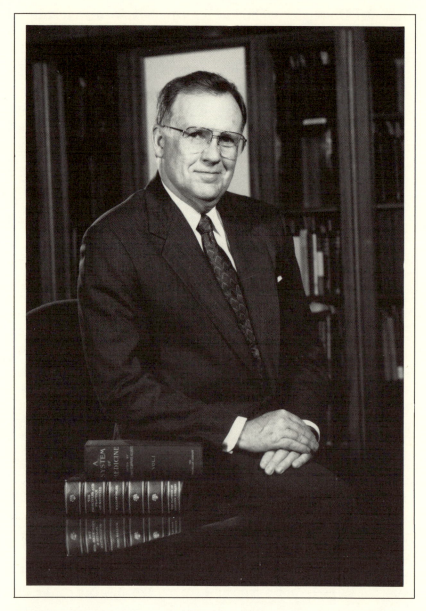

David M. Richards, D.O., who joined the college in 1981, has held the president's chair since 1986. His administration has been responsible for increasing admissions standards and enlarging community-service programs.

schools across the country. "This is an aspect of medicine and medical education that needs to be emphasized," says Ogilvie, founding chair of the department.

At TCOM the department embraces several disciplines: medical ethics; the history of medicine; medical jurisprudence. It includes the impact of art, language, literature and religion on medicine and has been responsible for a program of teaching medical Spanish so that physicians can communicate with patients who speak Spanish but not English. In cooperation with Texas Christian University, the department instituted a program in which medical students, divinity students and nursing students were team taught medical ethics.

One of the most effective programs established by the department of medical humanities was a series of evening lectures which brought recognized authorities on the history of medicine to the TCOM campus. Southwestern Medical School in Dallas had a similar program, and close cooperation developed between the two institutions: programs would be on one campus one year, the other the next.

TCOM's research program devoted to the principles behind the osteopathic profession is another unusual addition to traditional osteopathic education. Known as CORE (Center for Osteopathic Research and Education), the program grew out of recommendations of the task force which developed the educational goals statement.

I. M. Korr explains, "We had come to the conclusion that this was a college of osteopathic medicine and therefore the teaching of osteopathic medicine, its principles and its practice, its scientific foundation should be the responsibility of the entire college, every department." There was, in the early eighties, one department charged with teaching osteopathic theory and practice; the task force proposed yet a second team to look into making the entire college osteopathic.

Korr was named acting director, with a permanent director, an osteopathic physician, to be appointed later. "It was," says Korr, "recommended that the acronym, CORE, be used as a kind of imitation of my own name, and I appreciated that very much."

Today, President Richards charges CORE—and the department of manipulative medicine—with the responsibility for increasing scholarly activity in osteopathic research. "We know as practicing osteopathic physicians," he says, "that there are osteopathic or manipulative things that we can do for the patient with colon cancer, for instance—not necessarily to cure the cancer but to help that patient's total well-being during the process of therapy. But we need to produce research that provides a direct answer to that question; we can't simply expect students to believe us any more." Richards' eye is on double-blind studies with fields of three hundred patients or more, and papers published in prestigious medical journals. "We must have the data base," he says, and he predicts that, with CORE, TCOM will provide such a data base in the near future.

Despite the complexities of the clinical program at TCOM, the department of general and family practice remains central to the clinical experience of each and every student. "The department is central to our challenge to provide generalists who will provide health care particularly for the underserved populations in Texas," explains Dr. John Peckham, associate dean for primary care. "A lot of those underserved populations are in small towns. We've proven statistically that a high percentage of our graduates locate in communities with under a hundred thousand population and they are in primary care practices in these communities. The department of general and family practice is essential to that record."

The clinical program at TCOM continues to evolve, a blending of traditional medical education and innovative ideas and programs that speak to the health needs of this state and this country in the next century.

৪৪৪ *The Basic Science Program*

TRADITIONALLY, OSTEOPATHIC SCHOOLS HAVE HAD LITTLE EX-
ternal funding for research. TCOM, like most of its fellow institutions, began with insignificant amounts of funding. But in its twenty years of existence the college has put impossibilities to rest, establishing internationally recognized research programs in the basic sciences, with backing amounting to almost four million dollars.

The basic science teaching program really began in July of 1970, months before the school opened. Dean Henry Hardt asked Dr. Elizabeth Harris to prepare a budget, and after careful study, she came up with operating expenses of $75,900 (exclusive of faculty salaries) to teach anatomy, physiology, biochemistry and microbiology.

Faculty assignments were withheld until the curriculum was settled, and then it evolved that during the first semester Harris would teach embryology—she had previously taught the subject at Louisiana State University and had graduate experience in the field; Charles Rudolph taught biochemistry; and Tom Graham, cell physiology.

Mary Lu Schunder taught anatomy and enlisted the aid of various local specialists—when the subject of study was the head and neck, Ed Becka, an ENT specialist, lectured; a podiatrist spoke on the foot, and surgeons from FWOH were frequent lecturers. Harris recalls that general practitioner Bob Nobles of Denton gave the first lecture in anatomy, talking about things he wished he'd paid more attention to in medical school. "It was dynamic," says Harris, stressing that throughout those early basic science courses the emphasis was on the things students would need to remember as general practitioners.

Pathologists Gerald Bennett and Myron Skinner from the staff of FWOH taught histology, even preparing their own slides and arranging for students to view gross tissues in the hospital pathology lab. "Bennett would summon the students to see unusual pathology on the spot," says Elizabeth Harris. "Once it was a hydatid mole [aberrant pregnancy] and choriocarinoma [cancer of the placenta]. We stopped class and went to the lab, and Bennett lectured impromptu on the subject. It was great for the students."

The second semester immunology was added to the curriculum, and students took physiology instead of cell physiology. They studied both gross and neuroanatomy, which put an unbelievable strain on Schunder, the only anatomy instructor. At Harris' suggestion, Rudolph taught clinical biochemistry.

Harris cites the tremendous influence of internist Ray Olson on the basic science curriculum at the time. He encouraged the use of actual case histories—and actual patients—in immunology, and later in his introduction to medicine course he always called upon one of the basic scientists to present the background information on a case. Depending on the nature of the clinical problem, Schunder or Harris or Rudolph would give the scientific background. "It was an excellent course," Harris recalls.

By the second year of the college's operation, Bennett had left Fort Worth to work in Kansas City, and Elizabeth Harris was placed in charge of the general pathology course. She made assignments to various physicians and basic scientists. Feliks Gwozdz, M.D., the chief medical examiner for Tarrant County, agreed to come and give one lecture on cancer. "He had such a good time," says Harris, "that we [Elizabeth Harris, George Luibel and Carl Everett] took him to dinner and talked him into teaching systemic pathology." Gwozdz became so popular with the students that he and his family, all talented musicians, provided entertainment at every senior banquet from 1974, when the first class graduated, until 1980 when the pathologist's unexpected death ended the tradition.

Two more basic scientists had joined the faculty in 1971—Drs. John Gaugl in physiology and James Murphy in pharmacology. Along with the founding basic scientist faculty—Elizabeth Harris, Schunder, Rudolph, Graham and Banister—they carried far heavier teaching loads than would have been assigned in a school with a longer history. They had no time for independent research, generally the key to career advancement for basic scientists. Nor, until the opening of Med Ed II, did they have adequate equipment or laboratories. Asked if this was a professional sacrifice, Elizabeth Harris responds, "Certainly. It slows academic recognition. I'm an associate professor for life because of it, but I'd do it again any time."

Teaching and research programs in the basic sciences took a giant step in 1972 when the college first contracted with North Texas State Universty. The basic science programs were moved to the Denton campus, and TCOM sent one full-time faculty member from each of its basic science departments—biochemistry, anatomy, pharmacology, physiology and microbiology—to teach on the Denton campus. NTSU put ten faculty members into the program, most of whom had ongoing research projects underway, but the main teaching responsiblity still lay with TCOM faculty who had been transferred to the NTSU payroll.

"We already had full teaching loads," recalls Dr. Ben Harris, a member of the NTSU faculty at the time and now associate dean for research at TCOM, "but we were offered a summer salary to teach yet another course in the medical program." He explains that NTSU faculty then were paid on a nine-month program; in order to have summer income, they either had to teach a summer session or secure a research grant. The medical program offered faculty members a third option, but it added to an already heavy teaching and research load.

The funding that came with state affiliation, however, brought the biggest changes to the basic sciences program because the college was able to hire new faculty. "We gained critical mass in the basic sciences faculty," says Ben Harris. "The association with a

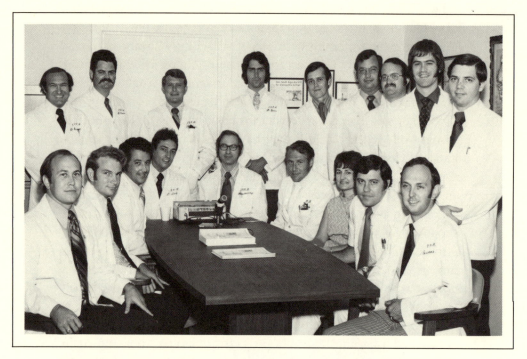

*The pioneering class of 1974: standing (left to right), Shelley M. Howell,
Gilbert E. Greene, Jobey D. Claborn, Sterling F. Lewis, R. Paul Livingston,
Weldon E. Bond, T. David Wiman, Robert G. Holston, and Jesse R.
Ramsey; seated, Ronald D. Sherbert, John H. Williams, Ronald L. Daniels,
Kenneth J. Brock, Robert J. Breckenridge, Terry L. Parvin, Nelda N.
Cunniff, David A. Ray, and John L. Sessions.*

medical school was important because it offered advantages like a twelve-month contract instead of nine months, better salary, good promise for the future. Graduates with degrees in biological and biomedical sciences usually choose between teaching in a university or a medical school, and there are advantages to each—a university is certainly a more relaxed atmosphere. But we were able to offer new faculty the combination, and that was a real plus."

Ben Harris mentions the department of biochemistry as a leader in developing programs and credits the strong direction of Dr. Robert Gracy who assumed the chair of that department in 1976. Gracy, says Harris, took control of the department with a positive approach and began recruiting faculty.

By the late seventies, laboratory space and equipment were available on the Fort Worth campus, and search committees began to look for additional faculty candidates with strong backgrounds in scholarly research. From 1976 until 1979, Dr. Gordon Skinner served as dean of basic sciences at TCOM, chair of the basic health sciences department at NTSU, and director of research at TCOM.

In 1981 when David Richards became dean for academic affairs, he saw a need to strengthen the college's research base. A select committee was appointed to explore the problem, to do an assessment of the college's resources in terms of faculty and its research needs as an institution. They formulated what is now known as the research goals statement. Among their recommendations: hire a dean of basic sciences and research. Ben Harris was appointed on an interim basis; today he serves as associate dean for research while Dr. Carl Jones is associate dean for the basic sciences. "The program took off," says Richards. "Our Ph.D. faculty had the experience, and they took off running."

"We began the eighties with under one million dollars in external research funding," says Ben Harris. "Today we are up to four million, and that's for a basic science faculty of forty-five members. There's an attitude of research, a real surge in scholarly activity." And with that surge came advances in the teaching program, as new faculty were imported and as the academic atmosphere stimulated the existing faculty.

Ben Harris cites several examples of internationally known research scientists on the faculty: Dr. Robert Gracy, who studies the biochemistry of aging and recently received a MERIT (Method to Extend Research in Time) grant from National Institutes of Health that will amount to about three million dollars over the next ten years—"you can't apply for these," explains Harris, "but they are granted with the application for an extension of research, based on past performance and the expectation of future performance"; Dr. Myron Jacobson, whose work is on the biochemistry of niacin (one of the B vitamins) in cancer and who organized an international symposium at TCOM in 1987 which was attended by 200 delegates from twenty-two countries; Dr. Harbans Lal of pharmacology who studies the effect of psychoactive drugs in memory decline; Dr. Peter Raven's studies in exercise physiology; or Harris' own studies in the biochemistry of parasitic worms. Research projects undertaken at TCOM are making a significant contribution to the international understanding of health.

With the basic science research program fairly well established, Ben Harris sees the biggest challenge in clinical research. "Our students get the best clinical teaching in the state because it's one on one, but that means the clinicians have no time for research. If we had a huge teaching hospital, the clinicians would have house staff which would free them for research activities."

One answer at TCOM is to encourage students to look at joint degrees, D.O./Ph.D. or D.O./M.S., with research training in their area of special interest—biochemistry, manipulation, toxicology, whatever. "We have to train our own scholars," says Harris. Chancellor Hurley agrees that these programs will provide the basic science and research leadership needed in osteopathic medical education.

Twenty years from now? "We'll be a full academic health sciences center with significant outside funding and an internationally known clinical faculty," he predicts. "We have internationally recognized people now in the basic sciences. We have to produce academically oriented clinicians."

Ben Harris sees no conflict between the college's focus on the training of general practitioners and his emphasis on academically oriented clinicians. In fact, he stresses the importance of academic specialists in training physcians to be generalists. "They must be taught by masters in each field, because they have to know the details of *everything*. They have to be taught biochemistry by a functioning biochemist, one who lives his biochemistry rather than just getting it out of a textbook."

Today, basic science faculty not only hold appointments at UNT but also hold joint appointments in clinical departments to assist in developing teaching and research. "Internal medicine, for example," says Richards, "is basically pathology, physiology and pharmacology. Cardiology research is closely related to physiology."

Community Service: A Tradition of Caring

IN THE FIRST YEARS OF THE COLLEGE, PEDIATRICIAN VIRGINIA Ellis took care of the students' children without charge. "I grew up at a time when all doctors took care of other doctors' families," she explains. "It's a basic sharing which goes on in this profession. . . . When you give to someone in this world, part of you is part of their lives. And it's just the same way when they do something for you— part of their lives belongs to you."

Ellis, the daughter of two practicing osteopathic physicians, absorbed the importance of community service from her parents. Traditionally, osteopathic medicine has been a service profession, and in Fort Worth the profession had a history of involvement in the community.

The local osteopathic auxiliary, for instance, sponsored an annual Child Health Clinic, based on models provided by the osteopathic communities in Amarillo, Texas, and Kansas City, Missouri. Physical examinations were offered to the children of the community, at first for free and later for one dollar per child. The former Texas Hotel in Fort Worth donated space, and various pharmaceutical companies helped to underwrite the cost of the clinic. Ellis remembers the first year: "We had no idea what to expect. We didn't know if any children would come, but all of the sudden there were children all over that hotel lobby. We were overrun."

Before the first TCOM students reached the clinical phase of their training, Ellis was carrying on the tradition of community service.

The Community Action Agency (CAA) asked her to work one morning a week at a well-baby clinic in a center on the east side of Fort Worth. Eventually, another local physician, Dr. Al Pressly, spelled her at the clinic, and they alternated Thursday mornings for a long time. In the third year of the college's operation, Ellis joined the full-time faculty, bringing with her her own personal tradition of community service.

In the 1972–73 academic year, which was the inaugural year of clinical training for the first class, a leader in the black community asked Ellis to bring students to the clinic. Eventually the clinic became part of the Headstart program and moved to the Bethlehem Clinic on Fort Worth's southeast side. In 1990, students still serve at the Bethlehem Clinic.

"The students love it," says Ellis. "At convocation this year [1989] two students came up and said they wanted to meet me because they knew I'd started the program at Bethlehem, and they just wanted me to know how much they learned from it, how important they felt it was."

In November 1973, the college also began its Mobile Clinic program. The Community Action Agency bought a van or recreational vehicle, and the college outfitted it with a treatment table and the bare essentials for emergency medical care. The van visited eight community action agencies for about three hours every two weeks—that meant that the van, with students and a supervising licensed physician, went out four days a week. The agencies made the appointments; the students and physicians saw the patients.

"Every year, I sent out a little questionnaire at the beginning of the year," recalls Ellis, "and I had three little things, so they only had to check one place and return it. One said, 'I'd be happy to drive the Mobile Unit.' Another said, 'I would, but I'd rather not.' And the third said, 'No way!' That was how I found my drivers.

"It was exciting," she says, "and it really served as a wedge into the community. But Dr. Newell convinced me that we couldn't do ongoing care visiting those clinics only once every two weeks, and we weren't doing enough episodic care to be a good teaching program. And that was what we were about first—teaching. The CAA ran out of money, and the Mobile Unit program was no more. But it was a tremendous experience while it lasted." The alternative was the outpatient clinics scattered throughout Fort Worth and surrounding rural communities. Essential to the clinical teaching program of the college, they operate also as community-service programs.

By the early eighties, Ellis was director of community services and oversaw a multi-faceted program which sent students to all kinds of community functions and locations—Mayfest, Oktoberfest, health fairs, marathons, shopping mall special events and the like. Dispensing emergency health care and educational advice, as the situation warranted, the college became a real presence in the community.

Ellis designed a community service program with emphasis on care of the aging, substance abuse, the handicapped and retarded, human sexuality, and death and dying. Students were required to choose three of the five topics for their program, and they met in traditional classroom situations to consider the topics. "Community support was fantastic," says Ellis, noting that people from all over the community came to teach when their topic was under consideration.

"A doctor is going to help patients, and he or she must realize the many things that contribute to health or disease," she says. "They've got to understand the importance of family situation, work status, all those things that go into the total person."

Ellis also believes that physicians do not need to know the answer to every question themselves. What they must know is where to go for help. "They've got to understand, for instance, that they can't cure an alcoholic. But they need to know where to send the alcoholic and where to send the family."

Accordingly, the community service curriculum worked with several agencies. Students were required, for instance, to attend a meeting of Alcoholics Anonymous. Other programs were elective, but they were offered the opportunity to visit Planned Parenthood, to work with Cenikor, the program for dealing with abuse of hard drugs, to attend a meeting of Tough Love, which helps disturbed teenagers and their families, and to visit the Moncrief Radiation Center and actually work with patients undergoing radiation therapy.

Today the community service program has been integrated into various clinical departments of the general education program, but it is a strong presence within the curriculum of the college because of the traditional osteopathic emphasis on community service and because of the programs developed by Ellis and her colleagues. The tradition of caring, she says, goes on and on.

The tradition of caring goes on in the community clinics operated by the department of general and family practice. Just as that department is central to the clinical program, the experience in a community clinic is central to the education of the TCOM student. Each fourth-year student spends three months in a general practice clinic; appropriately, it is the longest rotation in any discipline. In clinic rotations, students get their central experience in conducting their own general practice; for the many students who will become family physicians, practicing general osteopathic medicine, service in the community clinics gives them their first taste of their future professional lives. And most of them find the taste whets the appetite.

TCOM opened its first community clinic in July 1973. Located on Rosedale Avenue, it became known as the Rosedale Clinic. Ellis remembers early days there. "Dr. William A. Griffith was the director, and he just was really neat. The students liked him, and he liked his work. But he had to have a day off, so I supervised. . . . I had to assist with some real strange decisions, like how do you make out a list of supplies in the office?" The problems of organization at the clinic were eased somewhat when Edna Stokes transferred from the business office to the Rosedale Clinic as the first physicians' assistant.

The second clinic, known as Central Clinic, was opened in March 1974 adjacent to the administration building on Camp Bowie Boulevard.

Dr. Richard Baldwin was associate dean for clinical affairs in the late seventies when the outpatient clinic program was expanded.

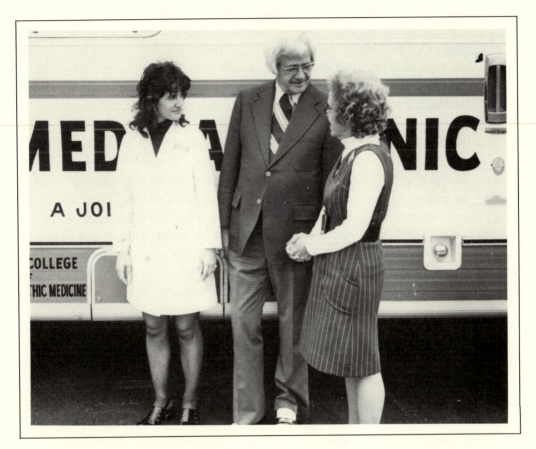

Nelda Cunniff, Dr. Ed Newell and Dr. Virginia Ellis in front of the mobile clinic.

He cites a bit of history to explain the need for expansion of the program. "In 1975, the college agreed to limit its enrollment to classes of seventy-three for three years but far greater class size was anticipated in the future. It was obvious that more clinics were needed to provide a volume of general practice for increased enrollment over the next few years."

The college took a decentralized approach to general practice clerkship education, although, as Baldwin says, "we could have done it all in one place. . . . We made an effort to go to areas of medical need," he says, "and build offices that were reasonably typical of what a doctor could expect to occupy in private practice in a small community. That, after all, is what we're about—training physicians to provide primary care in areas of need. The clinical rotation is training to get them comfortable in general practice."

The first rural clinic was opened in 1976 in Justin, a small town about thirty miles north of Fort Worth. Justin had a medical building, but the doctor who built it had been dead for ten years, and the town had had a series of doctors who stayed one or two years. When community leaders made overtures to TCOM, college officials thought Justin would be a good place for a new clinic.

In December 1976, the Northside Clinic was opened in Fort Worth's Northside Multipurpose Center. With the aid of federal money, the City of Fort Worth had funded a study to poll the Northside Hispanic neighborhood and say to the people, "What do you need?" The answer came back: a clinic, a daycare center, and a place where senior citizens can go for recreation and a hot meal at noon. The city built a multipurpose building to meet those three basic needs and asked the college to operate the clinic. All employees at that clinic and, when possible, students and faculty physicians, are bilingual.

A second rural clinic was opened in 1980 in Godley, south of Fort Worth. Like Justin, Godley is about a thirty minute drive from the campus, close enough that a student could attend classes in the morning and spend the afternoon in the clinic. Also, like Justin, Godley had no physician. "We wanted another rural clinic," says

Baldwin, "because that best represents us and our mission as an institution."

In 1979, the college had closed the Rosedale Clinic. It was located in a older home and the space was inadequate. To continue serving the black community in Fort Worth, TCOM rented space in a strip mall in the southeast part of the city and opened the Riverside Clinic, which operated from 1979 until 1987.

"It was a question of facilities," says Baldwin. "We still serve the Riverside population through our Southside Clinic."

In late 1978, when the college occupied its first major building, Medical Education I, Central Clinic was moved into that facility, and its previous quarters were given temporarily to the Tarrant County Medical Examiner. Today, Central occupies quarters on the second floor of Med Ed I and is one of the busier clinics.

Meanwhile, in 1982, the city built a duplicate multipurpose center on the near southeast side, and the college took over that clinic. By 1987, it was apparent that the Riverside Clinic was blossoming and there was some overlap between it and the Southside Clinic.

At about the same time, TCOM was offered rent-free space to operate a clinic for military retirees at Carswell Air Force Base. The North Central Texas area is home to approximately 140,000 military retirees, and the base draws them for shopping, recreation and medical care. The on-base medical facilities were not sufficient to care for retirees, and the establishment of the Carswell operation seemed an ideal solution for both the college and the base. Riverside Clinic was closed and its equipment moved to Carswell.

Each office has a supervising physician, and clinics with a heavier patient load have two or three licensed doctors. "With the excitement and drama of the hospital and particularly the emergency room," says Baldwin, "students tend to think the only pathology is in the hospital. In the clinics, we show them that ambulatory care is important. They see a lot of people with a lot of problems."

The clinics also implement the goals statement, helping students to see that ambulatory care catches a patient before the acute phase of a disease. The wellness-oriented concerns—lifestyle, nutrition, exercise and so on—cannot easily be implemented in the acute-care setting of the hospital, but they are a natural part of primary care in a clinic.

"We are an unusual college," says Baldwin, "in that the president and the dean for academic affairs and the associate clinical dean all have backgrounds in general practice. General practice has a real presence in our institution."

So does community service.

The Next Twenty Years . . . and After

TEXAS COLLEGE OF OSTEOPATHIC MEDICINE HAS MADE GIANT strides in twenty years. Some will tell you that it couldn't have happened without state affiliation; others will credit the people . . . or the buildings . . . or the osteopathic profession. Perhaps it is all those things, woven together and working together, that have made a major institution out of a school that began as an impossible dream and whose history is one of impossibilities made possible.

TCOM's history began with things that many would say should not have been—a volunteer faculty with little or no educational experience, lecturers reaching far beyond their field of competence to teach whatever needed to be taught, make-do in many areas. Were this happening today, in a college with a twenty-year history, it would be cause for concern. Seen though as the birth of a new college of osteopathic medicine, such daring and creativity testify only to the determination of the founding faculty.

The college's history has also been characterized by bold innovation—a goals statement that seemed almost to rebuke traditional medical education, clinical departments not usually established at major medical schools, an unusually strong community service component to the educational program. In their implementation phase, these programs were free-standing units; today, they have been woven into the fabric of traditional medical education, so that at TCOM the program is forever highlighted by a concern for wellness, an awareness of the importance of the humanities to the prac-

III

ticing physician, a recognition that in many ways community service defines a physician's role in the community. Because of the dreamers who dared take medical education in new directions, the educational program at TCOM is rich with threads not found in other medical schools.

Speaking from the perspective of his previous association with the United States Air Force Academy, Chancellor Al Hurley suggests that all new professional schools have problems that center in the tension between theory and practice. At TCOM, he says, the challenge has been to balance the academic background with the practical, to see that basic science knowledge is integrated into the clinical experience. In the developing school, such problems mean change—programs may develop independently, only to be absorbed into other areas as the college matures.

Suggesting that osteopathic medicine has a tradition of a necessarily narrow focus, Hurley maintains "it is time to adjust to changes in the world. The same problem exists in the military—you have people who are perfectly capable of moving airplanes around the sky, but they are not the kind of leaders you need in the Pentagon."

TCOM more than holds its own in traditional, academic medical circles while accomplishing the health care goals that it has set for itself. In 1990, TCOM has an enrollment of almost 400 students; by law, ninety percent of each class must come from Texas. About seventy percent of all practicing graduates stay in the State of Texas. In an era of increasing specializiation, almost three-fourths of TCOM's alumni are family or primary care physicians, and more than a third serve towns of 25,000 or less.

The future? According to TCOM President David Richards, the next twenty years will see TCOM develop significant programs with the University of North Texas which "will allow us to implement our master plan." The college will play a significant role in the economy of Fort Worth and Tarrant County and in training of physicians to provide health care in the State of Texas. There will be increased affiliations with other health-care agencies, such as the VA. "Consortiums of that kind create patients, and with more pa-

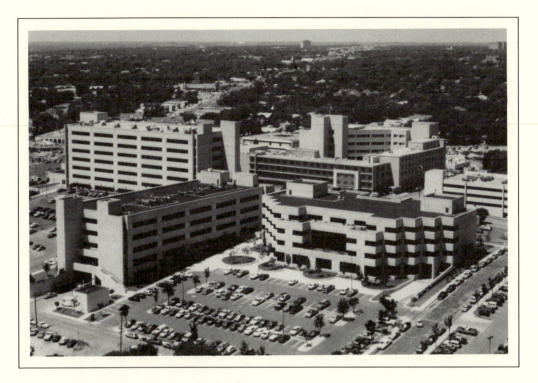

Texas College of Osteopathic Medicine, 1990.

tients to care for we can expand our programs. That leads to more faculty, and in turn more funding. The patient population is the key, and these affiliations provide those patients."

"TCOM has the challenge to provide important leadership to the osteopathic profession in the years ahead," says Hurley. "The need is not just for competent physicians but for broadly trained leaders for all fifteen of the osteopathic medical colleges, people who can keep renewing the profession. There are only a small number of qualified people—David Richards is unique is his background and capabilities—and we must focus on the younger people to develop those leadership qualities. TCOM students are highly qualified and they have that potential."

Both Hurley and Richards see continued emphasis on primary care as the central mission of the college. Perhaps Dr. T. Robert Sharp, former chairman of TCOM's scholarship and loan committee, says it best: "I would hope that the general practice image would be so polished as to stand as the emblem of what other ostepathic schools should be offering. . . . We have such a great [adjunct] faculty . . . all over Texas, and I would hope that we can keep an image of general practice both at our college here and . . . throughout the state."

At TCOM there are still many dreams to be made possible.

ᚼᚼ *Appendix*

Texas College of Osteopathic Medicine Sustainers

The following contributors, whose support of the college from 1969 to 1975 when TCOM was a private institution, are gratefully acknowledged for all to witness.

R. W. Anderson
D. R. Armbruster
M. E. Ayer
W. W. Bailes
J. E. Barnett
C. C. Bearden, Jr.
R. E. Beck
E. A. Becka
G. S. Beckwith
H. I. Benner
G. D. Bennett
M. F. Bennett
D. C. Benson
J. D. Bettis
H. L. Betzner
D. D. Beyer

R. B. Beyer
J. H. Black
R. A. Bowling
Russell B. Bunn
J. H. Burnett
Mary Burnett
H. G. Buxton
E. W. Cain
L. T. Cannon
M. A. Calabrese
Ruth E. Carter
G. J. Carlstrom
Catherine K. Carlton
J. C. Chapman
J. W. Coldsnow
M. L. Coleman, III

T. D. Crews
W. L. Crews
C. L. Curry
Palmore Currey
J. F. DePetris
C. E. Dickey
G. W. Diver
R. N. Dott
J. M. Dubin
D. L. Eakin
J. B. Eitel
H. F. Elliot
N. G. Ellis
H. A. Emory
C. E. Everett
L. D. Finch
R. B. Finch
Allen and Sue Fisher
Roy B. Fisher
J. E. Fite
L. F. Fite
W. V. Gabier
Sam B. Ganz
M. L. Glickfeld
Mrs. Russell Grace
H. G. Grainger
W. A. Griffith
O. E. Gutierrez
D. E. Hackley
R. M. Hall
R. G. Haman
R. L. Hamilton
Claude and Aldine Hammond
A. H. Hardy
D. H. Hause
E. A. Haynie

M. G. Holcomb
B. B. Jaggers
C. I. Jenkins
W. R. Jenkins
V. L. Jennings
J. D. Johnson
Mel E. Johnson
S. E. Jones
A. L. Karbach
J. C. Kemplin
E. C. Kinzie
Mrs. Vera Koetting
Arthur W. Kratz
M. G. Kumm
Casper Kutach
E. D. LaCroix
R. C. Leech
V. Mae and N. B. Leopold
R. A. Lester
C. H. Lewis
Mrs. Evelyn Lineberry
James W. Linton
J. L. Love
Laura A. Lowell
George J. Luibel
L. D. Lynch
S. G. Mackenzie
T. T. McGrath
A. Ross McKinney
Mrs. George F. McQueen
Carl Mitten
Mrs. Susie B. Neel
L. B. Nelson
R. H. Nobles
C. R. Olson
C. R. Packer

Pat Patterson
G. F. Pease
C. L. Perry
D. M. Peterson
R. H. Peterson
Mrs. R. H. Peterson
L. N. Pittman
E. P. Plattner
Hugo Ranelle
M. L. Richards
L. A. Wills
J. B. Riggs
Mrs. M. R. Roberts
W. B. Rountree
J. O. Royder
Phil R. Russell
W. R. Russell
P. Paul Saperstein
T. Robert Sharp
Bobby G. Smith
S. E. Smith
Marille Sparks

Sam Sparks
K. E. Speak
R. R. Stegman
R. L. Stratton
Wayne O. Stockseth
Joe Suderman
J. K. Taylor
D. T. Truitt
T. R. Turner
E. R. Tyska
R. C. Valdiva
A. W. Vila
R. L. Vinson
K. R. Watkins
F. S. Wheeler
Tom W. Whittle
A. S. Wiley
L. A. Wills
J. L. Witt
E. J. Yurkon
T. Eugene Zachary

❧❧❧ Index